5 Ingredients or Less Mini Instant Pot Cookbook

The Complete Instant Pot Duo Mini Recipes
Cookbook to Save Time and Money

By Heather Acevedo

Table of Content

Introduction

The instant pot has always been a great appliance to prepare some authentic and easy recipes without a lot of time, efforts, and fuss. The appliance needs a very little time to prepare food with much flavor and taste.

If you are a very busy person who could not find time to prepare some homemade food and get frustrated by long-standing and handle the overall food cooking process then this appliance best suited you. In less than 30 minutes you can cook even the hardest part of the meat to its tender perfection.

Most of the busy people are indulging in bad eating habits and prefer takeout options and junk food, which in return ruined their own physical health. But, with mini instant pot now anyone can prepare a hygienic and yummy food while carrying a busy schedule.

No doubt a mini instant pot is a trendy, latest, and multifunction appliance that consumes less electricity and time with more efficiency. But, as its name said it's not suited to prepare larger meals.

To get the better understanding of the appliance, let's start with some basic and detailed information in a few of the next chapters.

Chapter 1: Why You Must Have A Mini Instant Pot

Mini Instant pot is the latest appliance that actually combines a few of the kitchen appliance functions in one single device. It helps you to do anything from making rice, sautéing, steaming, and even making yogurt.

Mini Instant Pot is a small, affordable appliance that is designed by Canadians to provide convenience and safety at the same time. The mini instant pot speeds up cooking process 6 times and makes the food much healthier in nutritional content, by locking all the vitamins of the food.

There is not just a single reason to choose this appliance over any other appliance. You can prepare rice, soups, stews, yogurt, porridge, beans, cake and cookies using this mini device. It offers steam, sautéing, slow cooking, pressure cooking, and keep warm options. Build in programs helps you prepare food by simply pressing a single button.

You can also prepare side dishes and vegetables. It is a great appliance that covers a very less space and perfect for students, couples, and single person. It is so small in size that it can be accompanied during traveling.

The microprocessor that is built inside the mini instant pot is lab tested and uses an algorithm to control cooking time, temperature, and pressure. It helps in giving consistent results every time you prepare a new recipe.

The mini instant pot had a lid that fully sealed the appliance and locks the nutrients and aroma inside the meal; making it more healthy and delicious. Moreover, it keeps the environment odor free.

The heat is distributed evenly when cooking is done using mini instant pot. The pressure builds quickly inside the appliance; therefore minimal water is the need for cooking purposes.

The food cooked inside the mini instant pot retains its texture, color, and flavor, because of its remarkable consistency. No doubt, the mini instant pot is a versatile device designed to carter everyday needs.

The consistent results are provided because the mini instant pot is developed with 3rd generation technology that features an embedded microprocessor. The microprocessor monitors the pressure, time, heating, and duration of cooking during the cooking process. The volume of food is considered as well. The mini instant pot is no doubt a fully tested new technology that provides optimal and great tasting cooking experience.

Instant Pot continues to shock the user with its performance by making it easy to cook some healthy meals much faster.

What Is a Mini Instant Pot (3-Quart)?

The mini instant pot (3 quarts) is a device like all other instant pots; the difference is in its size. It is a 9-in-1 programmable device that replaces several appliances in the kitchen by providing nine functions of the slow cooker, steamer, cake maker, sterilizer, sauté, yogurt maker, rice cooker, warmer, and pressure cooker. It is a very versatile appliance that is used to prepare a home-based meal in small portions. The mini instant pot can cook up to 6 cups of rice. It comes with its own rice measurement cups, stainless steel racks, rice paddle, soup spoons, and condensation collector.

Amazing Benefits of Using a Mini Instant Pot

- It offers a one-touch technology for most of the common cooking tasks.
- It helps prepare food much faster than any other cooking method.
- It preserves the natural taste and nutrients of food.
- It offers a very easy and hand free cooking experience.
- The food is cooked at high pressure that kills any harmful micro-organisms.
- It offers a clean and pleasant cooking environment.
- It saves electricity and provides hustle free cooking.
- Its safety features make it one of the safest appliances to use. The pressure sensor technology helps regulate the pressure inside the cooker with much precision.
- If you don't want to spend money on different appliances to complete the several cooking tasks, then this device can work wonders for you by providing features of 7 appliances in one.

How to Choose a Perfect Mini Instant Pot?

Everyone chose an instant pot according to their own personal preferences, but it's crucial to keep in mind a few points before making a buying/choosing decision. The first question is which instant pot is right for you? There are a series of models available in the market that carter every person's individual needs. While choosing through the huge collection, size, and functions of instant pots, it sometimes gets very confusing.

Well, first you need to check for what purpose you are buying the instant pot. If you are interested in making side dishes, small meals, yogurt, stews, soups, then the mini instant pots are just for you. The mini instant pot is not suited and designed to prepare large portions of meals.

Do keep in mind that the pot when advertised about holding the volume to a certain limit, it usually means to the top, and no one fills a pot to the top, to make a mess. The room for expansion is needed. It should be kept in mind that what a 3 quart can hold. If you are a single person, then 3 is a good choice for you.

Where Can I Buy a Mini Instant Pot?

Instant pot mini can easily be purchased from retail stores and online stores like the Instant Pot Store and Amazon.

Chapter 2: Know about Its Features and Buttons

Features of the Mini Instant Pot (3 –Quart)

The appliance offers 11 smart buttons of soup/broth, meat/stew, rice, bean/chili, porridge, sauté, steam, yogurt, keep warm, slow cook, and pressure cook, to prepare some delicious dishes with a single touch. It has a user-friendly LED display, that shows cooking status. It also offers a dual pressure setting for the flexible cooking. Its high-pressure setting cooks the food 70 % faster, and the low setting ensures that the delicate items are not overcooked.

The adjustment settings are quick and easy to use. Instant pot mini is a very smart appliance as it remembers three sets of customization in each cooking program, that is more, less, and normal. The mini instant pot 3-quart can cook up to 4 hours at high pressure. Automatic keep warm option can keep the food stay warm for up to 10 hours. The mini instant pot 3-Quart came with stainless steel interior and brushed stainless steel exterior.

Some other feature includes:

- Dimensions: 11.81 x 10.51 x 11 inches
- Heating Element: 700 watts
- Power supply: 120V – 60Hz
- Weight: 8.65 pounds
- Power Supply Cord: 35 inches, detached, 3 prong plugs.

Mini Instant Pot Buttons

Which button is used to cook which food item? Is important to understand. The mini instant pot got following button that works with just a single click.

- Soup/Broth: The soup and broth button are used to prepare some delicious and mouth watering soup recipes.
- Porridge button: It is used to prepare some quick porridge.
- Meat and stew button: Meat and stew button is used to prepare some finest cut of meat to its tender perfection. It also offers stew making.
- Steam: Steam button is used to steam some delicious food items, by locking all the nutrients inside.

- Less, Normal or More function: This function is achieved by pressing the same cooking function button repeatedly to reach less, normal, or more according to personal preferences.
- (-)And (+) function button: It helps to adjust the cooking time by pressing up (+) or down (-).
- Bean/Chili: The button is used to cook beans and chilies
- Yogurt button: If you love yogurt making then this button help you prepare the yogurt with the most ease.
- Rice: It's used to cook rice. The button adjusts the time, according to the amount of rice and water added to the pot.
- Slow Cook: Its use to slow cook the desirable meal.
- Sauté: Once the sauté button is pressed, you need to wait until it reads "hot" on display; afterward you can add the ingredients to the pot. If you want to brown the meat, then adjust it to "more" setting.
- Cancel: End the cooking process.
- Delay: It helps the mini instant pot to start the cooking time after the amount of time is set for the delay.
- Pressure Cook: It is used for pressure cooking by choosing between high and low pressure and adjusting the time by selecting and switching between (+) and (-) button.
- Pressure Level function button: Help choose between high and low pressure for pressure cooking program. It works with all the buttons that cook at low or high.
- Keep Warm button: It helps keep the temperature inside the pot between 145 -170 degrees F.

A Brief Introduction of Different Cooking Methods

There are a few different cooking techniques that can be adapted to prepare some best tasting cakes, cookies, roasted meat, steamed vegetables, and much more.

Direct Cooking

The ingredients are directly cooked inside the inner Pot of the mini instant pot.

Pot in Pot Method

The PIP method helps you to pressure cook some of the best-tasting desserts, cookies, cakes, and cheesecakes, using a mini instant pot with ease and efficiency.

The Pot-in-Pot method allows the user to cook food in a separate bowl, which is placed on top of the rack or steamer basket. The rack is adjusted inside the instant pot, and the lid is sealed.

The food is pressure cooked, and after cooking time is over, the lid is opened after natural or quick release. The quantity this is being put in a separated bowl is less than what is cooked directly inside the pot. This process doesn't require any liquid added to the recipe, but the water is poured inside the pot, and then rack or steamer basket is adjusted on top. This method helps prepare all those recipes, that usually require baking. It includes Lasagna, meatloaf, cornbread, cookies, and cakes.

This method is also suited and perfect for a recipe that required Bain Marie; the technique that slow cook delicate recipes in the oven by steaming the dish to its perfection. The recipes like Creme Brulee, Dulce de leche, Savory custard, and Chocolate Lava Cake are perfectly made using this technique in the mini instant pot. The PIP method also helps to reheat the food or leftovers.

In the PIP method, the set of stackable containers also helps to cook multiple dishes at the same time. Multiple bowls can be stacked, separated by wire rack. This required the recipes to have the same cooking time, pressure levels, and pressure release method.

3 Quart Mini Instant Pot Vs Other Instant Pot

Models	DUO 60	DUO PLUS 30	DUO PLUS 60	DUO PLUS 80
Size	6 Quart	3 Quart	6 Quart	8 Quart
Dimension	13.4*12.2*12.5	11.4*10*11.2	13.4*12.2*12.5	14.8*13.3*14.2
Power				
Weight	11.8lbs	8.6lbs	11.84 Lbs	1561lb
Programmable Pressure Cooker	7 In1 (Slow Cooker, Pressure Cooker, Rice Cooker, Steamer, Sautéed, Yogurt Maker, Warmer)	9 In1 (Slow Cooker, Pressure Cooker, Rice Cooker, Steamer, Sautéed, Yogurt Maker, Warmer, Cake Maker, Sterilize)	9 In1 (Slow Cooker, Pressure Cooker, Rice Cooker, Steamer, Sautéed, Yogurt Maker, Warmer, Cake Maker, Sterilize)	9 In 1 (Slow Cooker, Pressure Cooker, Rice Cooker, Steamer, Sautéed, Yogurt Maker, Warmer, Cake Maker, Sterilize)
Delay Start Time	Yes	Yes	Yes	Yes
Keep Warm	Up To 10 Hours	Up To 24 Hours	Up To 24 Hours	Up To 24 Hours
Built-in Smart Programs				

Keep Warm	Yes	Yes	Yes	Yes
Sauté	Yes	Yes	Yes	Yes
Rice	Yes	Yes	Yes	Yes
Yogurt	Yes	Yes	Yes	Yes
Pressure Cook	Yes	Yes	Yes	Yes
Bean/Chili	Yes	Yes	Yes	Yes
Slow Cook	Yes	Yes	Yes	Yes
Multi-grain	Yes	No	Yes	Yes
Porridge	Yes	Yes	Yes	Yes
Cake	No	No	Yes	Yes
Sterilizer	No	Yes	Yes	Yes
Warm	Yes	No	No	No
Egg	Yes	Yes	Yes	Yes
Soup	Yes	Yes	Yes	Yes
Poultry	Yes	No	No	No
Meat/stew	Yes	Yes	Yes	Yes

Chapter 3: Most Useful Tips & Cautions of Using Mini Instant Pot

If you are an instant pot new user, then here are some tips and caution that needed to be followed for the better cooking experience.

Mini Instant Pot Cautions

- It is being recommended not to leave the home, while the instant pot is cooking. If it is really important to leave the home, then make sure that the steam is not coming out of the instant pot, and it had gone up to the pressure.
- It is absolutely not recommended for pressure frying the food.
- If the sealing ring is cracked or damaged, then it should be replaced.
- Once the cooking times complete for the specific recipe, use a quick release steam, or natural release steam to release the steam, and then open the pot.
- The thickening agents like the cornstarch or arrowroot powder should be added after the pressure cooking cycle has completed.
- The thick liquid produces less steam and pressure is not properly build, so it is important to adjust the thickness by adding water or stock.
- Use the sauté function to brown the meat.
- If you want to create a glaze of a cooked meal, then pour cold water into a hot inner pot, then scratch the sides and bottom, after taking out the food from the pot.
- It's not recommended to force open the pot.
- It's important to first make yourself sure about the steam is released fully. Once the pressure is released, the floating value drops.
- It's recommended to turn the setting knob to venting position to make sure all the pressure has been released.

Some Effective Tips

- To maintain the pressure the instant pot needs water or liquid, the liquid can be stock, vinegar, soup, or juice.
- Never fill the inner pot of the instant pot more than halfway, as while cooking, the food expands.
- It is very crucial to wash the inner pot, anti-block shield, lid, and the inner surface after every use.
- Before using the instant pot inspect the sealing ring that it is well sealed in the ring rack and the anti-block shield is mounted properly on steam release pipe.

- Never pull the sealing ring with a lot of force as it may lead to deformation and affect the function in sealing the pressure inside the pot.

Common Mistakes You Must Avoid

Here are some common instant pot mistakes that needed to be avoided:

- A lot of people make a mistake of not turning the pressure valve to sealing. You know that the mistake has been made when you hear a weird sound when the pressure has built inside the pot, or when the instant pot does not beep even the cooking times have completed. To avoid such flaws, it is important to make a habit of putting the lid, then closing it, and making sure that the valve is set to sealing. Do not press any button until the valve set correctly.

- Another common mistake is that the users not place the sealing ring back inside the lid. Make a habit of putting the sealing ring back at the same time when it is being taken out for cleaning purposes.

- If there is not enough water added to the pot the food gets burned while cooking. So always start by adding liquid, but it's also important to note that you cannot put a bunch of ingredients in the instant pot until the cooking cycle is done.

- You cannot cook all types of food by just adding them together and wait for a delicious meal to come out. Like rice and red meat has different cooking time and pressure level, so be sure while adopting such recipes use pot in pot method.

- Cooking and pressure level, both should be taken into account to prepare a meal perfectly.
- Use the right type of release option for the type of food, cooking in the pot. Like meat always benefit from the natural release option.

- Don't forget to turn off the warm button, as once the warm button is pressed the food will go on cooking and eventually can get overcooked.

Chapter 4: Maintenance of Mini Instant Pot and Some FAQs

Once you have bought a mini instant pot and start making some delicious treats, then you might also start to think that how to get rid of mini instant pot odor and discolored liner. Well, keeping the appliance clean, odor free and well maintained is crucial for its efficiency and durability. If you are looking for answers to these questions, you are in a right part of the book. This chapter will demonstrate step by step process to keep the appliance clean, odor free for fast and better performance and cooking experience.

How to Clean It (Step-By-Step)?

Step No 1: Cleaning the Exterior of the Instant Pot

Take a clean, damp cloth and wet it with water, then wipe off any residual on the outer surface of the instant pot. The microfiber cleaning cloths are recommended to do the job magically. Next, clean the rims of the mini instant pot with the help of a foam brush. After cooking the dripping and food items get caught in the rim, therefore foam brush is ideal to clean such complex parts of the instant pot.

Step No 2: Cleaning the Inner Pot

Next, wash the inner stainless steel pot with soapy warm water and rinse it under runny water. Usually, the inner pot is dishwasher safe, so the advantage of the dishwasher can be taken instead of hand washing. If you notice any discoloring or rainbow stain at the bottom, then don't get panic, as it can easily be solved by using white vinegar. Leave the inner pot with the spray for vinegar for a while to revive a fresh and shiny inner pot.

Step 3: Washing the Lid

Wash the lid of the instant pot with warm soapy water. It's not recommended to wash the lid in the dishwasher. Lift up the anti-blocking shield and then rinse and tap dry.
Pull the steam Release Valve to wash it under tap water Condensation Collector should be taken out and washed as well.

Step No 4: Wash the Sealing Ring of the Mini Instant Pot

The instant pot sealing ring is a very crucial part to maintain the pressure inside the pot. It is very important to take care of it. The sealing ring is usually dishwasher safe. It is important to avoid any stretching or deforming the sealing ring.

Troublesome

The most common problem that the instant pot users face is the instant pot did not come to pressure. It happens a lot and troubleshooting the problem gets very frustrating. Here are some basic reasons for this problem along with the solution to help users troubleshoot the main cause.

- Sometimes the Steam release handle is in the venting position. To solve this issue open the instant pot and check that if the liquid is enough. If the liquid evaporates too much the instant pot won't pressurize. Next close the mini instant pot with release handle in the venting position. As the instant pot contents are warm, so it allows the user to close it properly. Once it's been closed move the steam release handle to seal position.
- The sealing ring known as the gasket is not seated properly by the user. For that push the sealing ring down all around the ring rack and make sure it's seated properly. It should move and rotate around the ring rack.
- The Sealing ring is misplaced. For that adjusts the sealing ring.
- If the sealing ring expends too much, it won't seal properly. The point that is needed to be noted is the sealing ring expands as it heated. But once it's cold down, it goes back to its natural state. If it cools down and still it is expanded, then it needs to be refrigerated or run under cold water.
- The sealing ring has food stuck inside or has debris, and then it's important to make sure that no food stuck to the ring. It is very important to clean the sealing ring and even all the parts of an instant pot after or before start cooking the new meal.
- If the sealing ring is damaged, it needed to be replaced.
- If the instant pot power cord is loose, then it needs to be pushed all the way.
- If the float value is up and the display reads "ON" and no countdown timer has begun. Then users should wait a bit to let the timer begin. The float value locks the lid, but the pot may need some time to pressurize. If the food is frozen, then it takes a lot of time for the instant pot to pressurize.

FAQS

Q. What is the color of instant pot mini duos?
A. Its color is stainless steel and black.

Q. Why should user own a mini instant Pot?
A. It is a very smart and perfect appliance that can be used for cooking side dishes, rice, vegetables, and meat. It is a best-suited appliance for students, couples, and a single person. It can also be carried along as traveling. It emits no steam, smell, or heat.

Q. Can mini instant pot be used for canning?
A. No, it is not suitable for such preparations.

Q. Can the user use mini instant pot for deep frying?
A. Users cannot pressure fry in the cooker with oil.

Q. How many safety mechanisms are added in a mini instant pot?
A. A total of 10 safety mechanisms are part of the mini instant pot.

Q. Can a user place a mini instant pot on the stovetop while the burner is on?
A. It's not recommended to place a mini instant pot near gas stove or burner.

Q. Can a user use a sealing ring of another instant pot brand for own mini pot?
A. It's only recommended to use own and recommended sealing ring and not to us an unauthorized or unapproved ring.

Chapter 5: 10 Easy Breakfast Recipes

Cheesy Egg Bake

Cooking Time: 24 Minutes
Yield: 2 Servings

Ingredients

4 slices of bacon, chopped
1 cup of hash brown, frozen
4 eggs
1/8 cup of plain cow's milk
¼ cup cheddar cheese, shredded
Salt and black pepper, to taste

Directions

1. Chop the bacon strips into small pieces.
2. Turn on the sauté mode of the mini instant pot and add bacon.
3. Cook it for 2 minutes, and then add frozen hash brown to the mini instant pot.
4. Cook it for 2 more minutes.
5. Now, grease a heatproof container that fits inside the mini instant pot with oil spray.
6. Whisk eggs along with milk and cheddar cheese in a bowl.
7. Season it with salt and black pepper.
8. Now, pour the egg mixture into the greased container.
9. Add cooked bacon and hash brown to the greased container, and stir to combine all the ingredients well.
10. Clean the inner pot of the mini instant pot.
11. Pour one cup of water into the mini instant Pot and then adjust the trivet on top.
12. Place the heatproof container on top of a trivet and then lock the lid of the mini instant pot.
13. Cook on high pressure for 18 minutes.
14. Next, release the steam by the quick release method.
15. Open the pot and then serve the dish.

Nutrition Facts
Servings: 2
Amount per serving
Calories   603
% Daily Value*

Total Fat 39.4g 51%
Saturated Fat 12.6g 63%
Cholesterol 385mg 128%
Sodium 1363mg 59%
Total Carbohydrate 29.6g 11%
Dietary Fiber 2.5g 9%
Total Sugars 2.6g
Protein 31.5g
Vitamin D 33mcg 163%
Calcium 182mg 14%
Iron 3mg 15%
Potassium 805mg 17%

Breakfast Bread in an Instant Pot

Cooking Time: 20 Minutes
Yield: 2 Servings

Ingredients
1 teaspoon of baking soda
1-1/2 cups of all purpose flour
1 tablespoon of vegetable oil
½ cup of whole milk
Salt, pinch

Directions
1. Combine baking soda, all-purpose flour, and salt in a bowl.
2. Next, gently pour milk into the bowl and mix it by hand to make the dough.
3. Add in the oil and continue mixing until the dough doesn't stick to the hands.
4. Cover the dough with aluminum foil, and let it sit until it rises in size.
5. Take a heatproof pan that fits inside your mini instant pot.
6. Pour water into the instant pot and adjust rack inside the mini instant pot.
7. Now, transfer the dough to a heatproof pan, adjust the pan on top of the rack.
8. Close the lid of the pot and adjust the timer to 20 minutes manually.
9. Once the timer beeps, use the natural release method for 10 minutes, then quick release.
10. Open the pot and remove the bread.
11. Set it aside to get cooled off.
12. Once done, serve by slicing. Enjoy.

Nutrition Facts
Servings: 2
Amount per serving
Calories   324
% Daily Value*
Total Fat 9.4g   12%
Saturated Fat 2.6g   13%
Cholesterol 6mg   2%
Sodium 732mg   32%
Total Carbohydrate 50.5g   18%
Dietary Fiber 1.7g   6%
Total Sugars 3.4g
Protein 8.4g
Vitamin D 24mcg   122%
Calcium 78mg   6%
Iron 3mg   16%
Potassium 154mg   3%

Pressure Cooker Scotch Eggs

Cooking Time: 15 Minutes
Yield: 1 Serving
Ingredients
2 large eggs, whole
½ pound of ground sausage, country style
½ tablespoon vegetable oil
Directions
1. Take a mini instant pot and pour water into it.
2. Now adjust a steaming rack in the pot and place eggs on top for cooking.
3. Set a timer for 5 minutes at high pressure.
4. Once the cooking time completes, release the pressure naturally for 5 minutes, then quick release the steam. Remove the lid of the pot and take out the eggs.
5. Put the eggs in cold water and remove the shells.
6. Next step is to divide the sausage into two equal proportions.
7. Flatten the sausage and place each piece of egg in the middle of the flat surface of the sausage. Gently wrap the egos with the sausage and make round balls.
8. Once eggs are wrapped, turn on the sauté mode of the instant pot and heat vegetable oil in it.
9. Now place the wrapped egg into the pot and cook for 5 minutes or until brown.
10. Remove the eggs from the instant pot.To the same pot, add water and place rack inside it.
11. Place the scotch eggs on the rack and then lock the instant pot with lid.
12. Cook on high pressure for 5 minutes. When timer beeps, quick release the steam.
13. Remove the eggs from the pot and serve.

Nutrition Facts
Servings: 1
Amount per serving
Calories   972
% Daily Value*
Total Fat 81.1g   104%
Saturated Fat 25.1g 126%
Cholesterol 563mg 188%
Sodium 1839mg   80%
Total Carbohydrate 0.8g   0%
Dietary Fiber 0g   0%
Total Sugars 0.8g
Protein 56.7g
Vitamin D 35mcg   175%
Calcium 83mg   6%
Iron 5mg   27%
Potassium 801mg   17%

Chocolate Steel Cut Oats

Cooking Time: 10 Minutes
Yield: 2 Servings

Ingredients
1 cup steel cut oats
2 small bananas, peeled
2 tablespoons of cocoa powder
2 cups of non-dairy milk
2 tablespoons of brown sugar

Directions
1. Place oats, milk, sugar, and cocoa powder into the mini instant pot.
2. Stir the ingredients well.
3. In a bowl, mash the bananas with a fork, and make a puree.
4. Now transfer the mashed bananas to the pot on top of all the ingredients.
5. Do not stir it.
6. Now close the pot and set the timer to 10 minutes at high pressure.
7. Once the timer beeps, release the steam naturally.
8. Remove the lid of the mini instant pot and stir the oatmeal.
9. Add more milk if like runny texture.
10. Enjoy.

Nutrition Facts
Servings: 2
Amount per serving
Calories   391
% Daily Value*
Total Fat 7.2g   9%
Saturated Fat 1.5g   7%
Cholesterol 0mg   0%
Sodium 132mg   6%
Total Carbohydrate 72.6g   26%
Dietary Fiber 9.4g   33%
Total Sugars 29.6g
Protein 14.5g
Vitamin D 1mcg   6%
Calcium 340mg   26%
Iron 5mg   26%
Potassium 657mg   14%

Instant Pot Breakfast Casserole

Cooking Time: 10 Minutes
Yield: 2 Servings
Ingredients
½ cup white onion, sliced
1 cup bell peppers green and sliced
1 tablespoon of olive oil
4 eggs
Salt and pepper, to taste
2 avocados, for garnish
Directions
1. Turn on the sauté mode of the instant pot.
2. Add olive oil to the pot and heat it up.
3. Add in the onions and bell peppers, and sauté for 4 minutes.
4. Turn off the instant pot and then transfer the ingredients to a heatproof soufflé pan that fit inside the mini instant pot.
5. Adjust a trivet inside the instant pot and pour a cup of water.
6. Now, crack the eggs on top of the peppers.
7. Sprinkle salt and pepper and then cover the pan with foil.
8. Make a sling of aluminum foil and then lower the soufflé pan on top of the trivet inside the instant pot
9. Lock the instant pot and cook it on high for 5 minutes.
10. Use the manual function to cook. Release the pressure quickly.
11. Remove the soufflé pan from the instant pot.
12. Serve by topping it with avocado. Serve and enjoy.

Nutrition Facts
Servings: 2
Amount per serving
Calories   213
% Daily Value*
Total Fat 16g 20%
Saturated Fat 3.8g   19%
Cholesterol 327mg   109%
Sodium 127mg   6%
Total Carbohydrate 6.9g   3%
Dietary Fiber 1.9g   7%
Total Sugars 3.7g
Protein 12.1g
Vitamin D 31mcg   154%
Calcium 61mg   5%
Iron 2mg   11%
Potassium 293mg   6%

Instant Pot Quinoa Breakfast Bowl

Cooking Time: 1 Minute
Yield: 2 Servings

Ingredients
1-1/2 cups white quinoa
1-1/2 cups water
1 cinnamon stick
1/4 cup raisins
1 tablespoon honey
1/3 cup apple juice

Directions
1. Rinse the quinoa under the water, and then add to the instant pot along with water, and cinnamon stick.
2. Then lock the lid.
3. Cook for one minute at high pressure.
4. Once the timer beeps, release the steam naturally for 10 minutes.
5. Then does a quick release steam.
6. Spoon out the quinoa to a medium bowl and then remove the cinnamon stick.
7. Add the honey, raisins, and apple juice.
8. Stir all the ingredients to combine well.
9. Refrigerate it for few hours before serving.
10. Enjoy with a dollop of a Greek yogurt as a side serving if liked.

Nutrition Facts
Servings: 2
Amount per serving
Calories   193
% Daily Value*
Total Fat 1.4g   2%
Saturated Fat 0.2g   1%
Cholesterol 0mg   0%
Sodium 9mg 0%
Total Carbohydrate 43.1g   16%
Dietary Fiber 2.9g   10%
Total Sugars 23.4g
Protein 3.7g
Vitamin D 0mcg   0%
Calcium 38mg   3%
Iron 2mg   10%
Potassium 189mg   4%

Egg Casserole in Instant Pot

Cooking Time: 7 Minutes
Yield: 2 Servings

Ingredients

4 eggs, whisked
4 tablespoons of milk
Salt and black pepper
2 tablespoons of chicken meat, chopped
¼ cup of cheese
2-4 Bread slices, as needed

Directions

1. Combine eggs, milk, meat, salt, and black pepper in a bowl.
2. Once all the ingredients are mixed up well, transfer to the ramekin that fits inside the mini instant pot.
3. Adjust a trivet inside a pot and pour a cup of water.
4. Place ramekins on top of the trivet and close the pot.
5. Adjust the timer to 7 minutes at high pressure.
6. Once it's done naturally release the steam and then opens the lid.
7. Remove the ramekin safely from the pot.
8. Let it sit for 2 minutes, then serve on your plate and top it off with cheese.
9. Place it on the bread slices and enjoy.

Nutrition Facts

Servings: 2
Amount per serving
Calories   239
% Daily Value*
Total Fat 15g 19%
Saturated Fat 6.3g   32%
Cholesterol 352mg   117%
Sodium 294mg   13%
Total Carbohydrate 6.9g   3%
Dietary Fiber 0.2g   1%
Total Sugars 2.5g
Protein 18.8g
Vitamin D 33mcg   163%
Calcium 200mg   15%
Iron 2mg   12%
Potassium 180mg   4%

Mini Instant Pot Bacon Ranch Potatoes

Cooking Time: 14 Minutes
Yield: 1 Serving

Ingredients
2 red potatoes, scrubbed and peeled and chopped
4 bacon strips
1 teaspoon dried parsley
Salt, to taste
½ teaspoon garlic powder
¼ cup Ranch dressing
3 tablespoons of water

Directions
1. Cut the potatoes into small pieces about 1 inch.
2. Chop the bacon strips into small pieces as well.
3. Turn on the sauté mode of the instant pot and cook bacon for about 2 minutes.
4. Next, stir in the potatoes and along with parsley, garlic powder and salt.
5. Now add water about few teaspoons.
6. Set the mini instant to manual for about 12 minutes at high pressure.
7. After 12 minutes quick release the steam.
8. Open the pot carefully.
9. Now add the ranch dressing.
10. Stir to combine well. Serve and enjoy.

Nutrition Facts
Servings: 1
Amount per serving
Calories   328
% Daily Value*
Total Fat 1.1g   1%
Saturated Fat 0.2g   1%
Cholesterol 2mg   1%
Sodium 577mg   25%
Total Carbohydrate 72.2g   26%
Dietary Fiber 7.5g   27%
Total Sugars 6.2g
Protein 9.9g
Vitamin D 0mcg   0%
Calcium 57mg   4%
Iron 3mg   19%
Potassium 1975mg 42%

Instant Pot Cornmeal Porridge

Cooking Time: 6 Minutes
Yield: 1 Serving

Ingredients

1 cup water, separated
½ cup milk
½ cup yellow cornmeal
1 stick of cinnamon
4 pimento berries
¼ cup sweetened condensed milk

Directions

1. Turn on the instant pot by pressing porridge button and setting it for 6 minutes.
2. Add half water and milk to the instant pot
3. Take a separate bowl and combine cornmeal with reserved water.
4. Mix well, and then add the cinnamon stick.
5. Now transfer it to the pot and cook for 6 minutes.
6. Once the cooking is done, release the steam naturally and then uncover the pot.
7. Add condensed milk and berries.
8. Mix well and then enjoy.

Nutrition Facts

Servings: 1
Amount per serving
Calories   542
% Daily Value*
Total Fat 11.4g   15%
Saturated Fat 6g   30%
Cholesterol 36mg   12%
Sodium 183mg   8%
Total Carbohydrate 98.4g   36%
Dietary Fiber 6.2g   22%
Total Sugars 48.8g
Protein 15.2g
Vitamin D 1mcg   3%
Calcium 399mg   31%
Iron 3mg   14%
Potassium 556mg   12%

Goji Berry and Oats Recipe

Cooking Time: 10 Minutes
Yield: 1 Serving

Ingredients

½ cup gluten-free rolled oats
1 cup almond milk or coconut milk
1/4 cup coconut cream
¼ cup Goji berries
2 tablespoons of   flaxseed
Pinch of sea salt

Directions

1. Pour the milk into the instant pot and add the oats, barley mix the ingredients and then lock the lid of the instant pot.
2. Cook on high pressure for 10 minutes.
3. Then release the steam naturally.
4. Once cooked, add in coconut cream, Goji berries, salt, and flaxseed.
5. Spoon out the oats and serve hot.
6. Enjoy.

Nutrition Facts

Servings: 1
Amount per serving
Calories   950
% Daily Value*
Total Fat 73.4g   94%
Saturated Fat 60.6g 303%
Cholesterol 0mg   0%
Sodium 296mg   13%
Total Carbohydrate 69.5g 25%
Dietary Fiber 12.2g 44%
Total Sugars 42.9g
Protein 12.5g
Vitamin D 0mcg   0%
Calcium 56mg   4%
Iron 12mg   64%
Potassium 806mg   17%

Chapter 6: 10 Delicious Poultry & Seafood Recipes

Ranch Chicken Chili

Cooking Time: 15 Minutes
Yield: 2 Servings

Ingredients

8 ounces of white chili beans, not drained
5 ounces of Rotel tomatoes and green chilies, not drained
½ ounce of taco seasoning
½ ounce of ranch seasoning mix
0.75 pounds of chicken breast, cubed

Directions

1. Combine the white chili bean, Rotel, taco seasoning, and the ranch seasoning in a bowl.
2. Add the chicken breasts to the bowl and mix well.
3. Dump all the ingredients in an instant pot and then cook on high pressure for 15 minutes.
4. Does a quick release steam, then serve and enjoy.

Nutrition Facts
Servings: 2
Amount per serving
Calories   365
% Daily Value*
Total Fat 11.3g   15%
Saturated Fat 3.1g   16%
Cholesterol 130mg   43%
Sodium 2070mg   90%
Total Carbohydrate 16.9g   6%
Dietary Fiber 5.6g   20%
Total Sugars 3.1g
Protein 44g
Vitamin D 0mcg   1%
Calcium 82mg   6%
Iron 5mg   27%
Potassium 1063mg 23%

Chicken for Tacos

Cooking Time: 24 Minutes
Yield: 2 Servings
Ingredients
2 pounds of chicken drumsticks, skin-on
1/3 cup balsamic vinegar
1/4 cup honey
½ cup soy sauce
4 cloves of garlic, minced
Salt and Black Pepper, to taste
Directions
1. Take a small bowl and combine together vinegar, salt, pepper, soy sauce, honey, and garlic.
2. Pour this sauce into the instant pot.
3. Place chicken drumsticks on top of the sauce and push it down, so the chicken submerges in the sauce.
4. Cook on high pressure for 20 minutes.
5. Once the cooking time completes, let the steam release, using the quick release method.
6. Now, turn on the sauté button so that the sauce boils and get reduced.
7. Now, place the drumsticks on parchment paper.
8. Preheat the oven to 350 degrees F.
9. Place the chicken inside the oven to broil for 4 minutes.
10. Then remove the chicken from the oven and transfer to the platter.
11. Pour the instant pot sauce over the top.
12. Serve and enjoy over tacos if liked.

Nutrition Facts
Servings: 2
Amount per serving
Calories   947
% Daily Value*
Total Fat 26g 33%
Saturated Fat 6.9g   34%
Cholesterol 399mg   133%
Sodium 3961mg   172%
Total Carbohydrate 42.2g   15%
Dietary Fiber 0.7g   3%
Total Sugars 36.1g
Protein 129.3g
Vitamin D 0mcg   0%
Calcium 78mg   6%
Iron 8mg   43%
Potassium 1117mg 24%

Instant Pot Curried Lemon Coconut Chicken

Cooking Time: 25 Minutes
Yield: 2 Servings
Ingredients
½ cup coconut milk
¼ cup of lemon juice
1 tablespoon of curry powder
Salt and black pepper, to taste
1.5 pounds chicken breasts or thighs
½ teaspoon of lemon zest
Directions
1. Combine coconut milk, lemon zest, lemon juice, curry powder, salt and black pepper in a bowl and mix well.
2. Now pour this mixture into the bottom of the mini instant pot.
3. Add the chicken thighs to the pot, stir ingredients well.
4. Now, set the timer to 25 minutes at high pressures.
5. Lock the lid and close the valve.
6. After the cooking cycle complete, use the quick release and open the pot.
7. Observe the chicken for doneness and then use the fork to shred the chicken inside the pot.
8. Mix all the ingredients well.
9. Serve with steamed rice and roasted vegetable of your choice.
10. Enjoy.

Nutrition Facts
Servings: 2
Amount per serving
Calories   802
% Daily Value*
Total Fat 40.2g   52%
Saturated Fat 19.9g 100%
Cholesterol 303mg   101%
Sodium 309mg   13%
Total Carbohydrate 5.9g   2%
Dietary Fiber 2.5g   9%
Total Sugars 2.8g
Protein 100.5g
Vitamin D 0mcg   0%
Calcium 78mg   6%
Iron 6mg   34%
Potassium 1073mg 23%

Chicken and Rice Congee

Cooking Time: 35 Minutes
Yield: 1 Serving

Ingredients

90 grams of rice, brown
2 cups cold water
2 chicken drumsticks
½ tablespoon ginger, sliced into strips
Salt, to taste

Directions
1. First, rinse the rice under tap water by gently scrubbing the rice.
2. Drain any milky water.
3. Next step is to add ginger, rice, chicken drumsticks, and water to the instant pot.
4. Do not add salt at this stage.
5. Now close the lid of the pot and cook on high pressure for 30 minutes.
6. Then, naturally release the steam.
7. Open the lid carefully; check if the congee looks watery.
8. Heat up the instant pot by pressing sauté button.
9. Cook until desired thickness is obtained.
10. Season it with salt and then use a fork to separate the meat from the bone.
11. Remove the congee from the pot.
12. Serve and enjoy.

Nutrition Facts
Servings: 1
Amount per serving
Calories   493
% Daily Value*
Total Fat 6g   8%
Saturated Fat 1.6g   8%
Cholesterol 81mg   27%
Sodium 248mg   11%
Total Carbohydrate 73.9g   27%
Dietary Fiber 1.5g   5%
Total Sugars 0.2g
Protein 32g
Vitamin D 0mcg   0%
Calcium 53mg   4%
Iron 5mg   30%
Potassium 328mg   7%

Stuffed Chicken

Cooking Time: 25 Minutes
Yield: 2 Servings
Ingredients
4 chicken breasts, boneless, skinless (butterfly cut)
½ cup frozen spinach
1/3 cup feta cheese, crumbled
Salt, divided
1/4 teaspoon of black pepper
1/4 teaspoon of garlic powder
2 tablespoons of coconut oil
1 cup Water
Directions
1. Pound the chicken breast pieces into 1/4 inch thickness.
2. Butterfly cut the chicken pieces and set aside for further use.
3. Take a medium bowl and mix spinach, feta cheese, pepper, garlic, and salt.
4. Divide this mixture evenly by spooning into the chicken breasts.
5. Close the chicken breast and secure with a toothpick.
6. Now, turn on the sauté mode of the instant pot and then add coconut oil to it.
7. Sear the chicken breast in batches until golden brown.
8. Then press the cancel button of the pot.
9. Set aside the chicken and go for next steps.
10. Now pour the water in the same pot and scrape the bottom to remove the seasoning.
11. Now adjust the steamer rack in the pot and place chicken on top of the rack.
12. Adjust the timer to 15 minutes at high pressure.
13. Once the timer goes off, naturally release the steam. Serve the dish hot.

Nutrition Facts
Servings: 2
Amount per serving
Calories   742
% Daily Value*
Total Fat 40.6g   52%
Saturated Fat 21.5g 107%
Cholesterol 282mg 94%
Sodium 617mg   27%
Total Carbohydrate 1.7g   1%
Dietary Fiber 0.3g   1%
Total Sugars 1.1g
Protein 88.3g
Vitamin D 0mcg   0%
Calcium 180mg   14%
Iron 4mg   22%
Potassium 775mg   16%

Dill and Lemon Salmon

Cooking Time: 5 Minutes
Yield: 2 Servings

Ingredients

2 salmon fillets (3 ounces each)
2 tablespoons of fresh dill, chopped
Salt and black pepper, to taste
1 cup Water
2 tablespoons of lemon juice
½ lemon, sliced

Directions

1. Sprinkle the salmon with dill, salt, and black pepper.
2. Place a steamer rack in the mini instant pot and pour one cup of water.
3. Place the salmon on top of the rack, skin side down.
4. Now drizzle lemon juice over the file and top each salmon with a slice of lemon.
5. Press the steam button and adjust the timer to 5 minutes, and close the lid of the pot.
6. Once done, quick release the steam.
7. Use the meat thermometer to make sure the internal temperature is 145 degrees.
8. Serve and enjoy.

Nutrition Facts
Servings: 2
Amount per serving
Calories   251
% Daily Value*
Total Fat 11.3g   14%
Saturated Fat 1.7g   9%
Cholesterol 78mg   26%
Sodium 92mg   4%
Total Carbohydrate 3.4g   1%
Dietary Fiber 0.9g   3%
Total Sugars 0.7g
Protein 35.4g
Vitamin D 0mcg   0%
Calcium 127mg   10%
Iron 3mg   15%
Potassium 827mg   18%

Garlicky Mussels

Cooking Time: 5 Minutes
Yield: 1 Serving

Ingredients

4 tablespoons of   butter, salted
4 cloves garlic, minced
1 pound mussels scrubbed and de-beard
1 cup chicken broth
1 tablespoon of lemon juice

Directions

1. Turn on the sauté mode of instant pot and melt butter in it.
2. When the butter melts, add in the garlic and sauté for 2 minutes.
3. Transfer the mussels in the mini instant pot and then add in the broth and lemon juice.
4. Press the cancel button to stop the sautéing.
5. Now close the lid of the instant Pot.
6. Now press the manual button and set the cooking time to 2 minutes.
7. Once the timers go off, release the steam using the quick release method.
8. Discard the unopened mussels.
9. Now transfer the cooked mussels from the instant pot to the serving bowl.
10. Pour the liquid from the mini instant pot on top.
11. Serve and enjoy.

Nutrition Facts
Servings: 1
Amount per serving
Calories   857
% Daily Value*
Total Fat 57.8g   74%
Saturated Fat 31.6g 158%
Cholesterol 249mg 83%
Sodium 2393mg   104%
Total Carbohydrate 22g   8%
Dietary Fiber 0.3g   1%
Total Sugars 1.2g
Protein 60.2g
Vitamin D 32mcg   159%
Calcium 164mg   13%
Iron 19mg   104%
Potassium 1739mg 37%

Instant Pot Shrimp

Cooking Time: 3 Minutes
Yield: 2 Servings

Ingredients

1 pound of shrimp
2 tablespoons butter, salted
½ tablespoon garlic, minced
¼ cup chicken stock
1-1/2 cup of cooked or boiled rice
Salt and black pepper, to taste

Directions

1. Turn on the sauté mode of the instant pot and add butter and garlic to it.
2. Once the butter melts and garlic turns brown, add the chicken stock.
3. Then add in the shrimp.
4. Cover the pot and turn off the sautéing mode.
5. Set the stew for one minute and then naturally release the steam for 5 minutes, then quick release the steam.
6. At this stage add the cooked rice to the pot and season it with salt and pepper.
7. Stir to mix well, and then serve.
8. Enjoy.

Nutrition Facts
Servings: 2
Amount per serving
Calories   713
% Daily Value*
Total Fat 16.1g   21%
Saturated Fat 8.7g   43%
Cholesterol 508mg   169%
Sodium 736mg   32%
Total Carbohydrate 78.2g   28%
Dietary Fiber 1.3g   4%
Total Sugars 0.2g
Protein 58.6g
Vitamin D 8mcg   40%
Calcium 241mg   19%
Iron 5mg   26%
Potassium 505mg   11%

Steamed Fish with Miso Butter

Cooking Time: 5 Minutes
Yield: 2 Servings

Ingredients
1 cup water
3 cloves of garlic, peeled
2 white fish tilapia fillets (about totaling 12 ounces)
Salt and Pepper, to taste
2 tablespoons of butter, melted
2 teaspoons Miso paste
2 tablespoons of soy sauce

Directions
1. Pour water into the instant pot.
2. Then add garlic and place trivet inside the pot covered with aluminum foil.
3. Place the fish on top of the foiled trivet, and drizzle soy sauce on top.
4. Then season fish with salt and pepper.
5. Close the pot lid and cook fish for 5 minutes at high pressure.
6. Meanwhile, make the Miso paste by mixing it with butter in a small separate bowl.
7. Set it aside for further use.
8. Once the fish is cooked, release the steam naturally.
9. Carefully remove the fish and then set aside.
10. Serve it with Miso butter paste.
11. Enjoy warm.

Nutrition Facts
Servings: 2
Amount per serving
Calories   687
% Daily Value*
Total Fat 18g 23%
Saturated Fat 10.1g 50%
Cholesterol 361mg 120%
Sodium 1442mg   63%
Total Carbohydrate 4.3g   2%
Dietary Fiber 0.5g   2%
Total Sugars 0.7g
Protein 128.2g
Vitamin D 8mcg   40%
Calcium 142mg   11%
Iron 7mg   41%
Potassium 70mg   1%

Salmon Relish

Cooking Time: 7 Minutes
Yield: 2 Servings

Ingredients
1 cup Water
2 salmon fillets, center-cut, (6-ounces each)
2 tablespoons grape seed oil or canola oil, divided
 Salt and black pepper, to taste
1 tablespoon tamari sauce
½ tablespoon sherry vinegar
½ teaspoon honey

Directions
1. Pour water into the instant pot and place steaming rack on top.
2. Cover the top of the rack with aluminum foil.
3. Brush the salmon fillet with half of the grape seeds oil.
4. Season the filets with salt and pepper.
5. Place the fish on top of foil on the steaming rack.
6. Press the steam button and set the timer to 7 minutes.
7. Once time completes, press cancel. Release the steam quickly.
8. Transfer the fish to the plate.
9. Now make a relish by mixing a tamari sauce, sherry vinegar, and honey in a bowl. Then add in the remaining oil as well.
10. Now spoon the sauce over the salmon and then serve. Enjoy.

Nutrition Facts
Servings: 2
Amount per serving
Calories   370
% Daily Value*
Total Fat 25g 32%
Saturated Fat 2.6g   13%
Cholesterol 78mg   26%
Sodium 585mg   25%
Total Carbohydrate 2g   1%
Dietary Fiber 0.1g   0%
Total Sugars 1.6g
Protein 35.5g
Vitamin D 0mcg   0%
Calcium 68mg   5%
Iron 1mg   8%
Potassium 705mg   15%

Chapter 7: 10 Mouth-watering Beef, Pork & Lamb Recipes

Instant Pot Barbecue Ribs

Cooking Time: 25 Minutes
Yield: 2 Servings
Ingredients
1 pound country-Style Loin Ribs
2 tablespoons barbecue meat rub, any personal favorite brand
1/3 cup vegetable broth
¼ cup apple juice
¼ cup barbecue sauce
Directions
1. The first step is to remove the membrane from the back of the rib.
2. Rub the meat with the meat, rub and then place it inside the instant pot.
3. Next, add the vegetable broth, and apple juice.
4. Close the lid of the pot and then cook on the manual mode by setting the timer for 20 minutes.
5. When the time is over, let the pressure release naturally.
6. It would take about 7-10 minutes.
7. Now remove the lid of the pot and then take out the ribs. Now, preheat the broil.
8. Transfer the cooked ribs to the baking sheet.
9. Brush the rib with BBQ sauce. Broil it for 5 minutes.
10. Once the sauce is caramelized, serve.

Nutrition Facts
Servings: 2
Amount per serving
Calories   841
% Daily Value*
Total Fat 57.8g   74%
Saturated Fat 21g   105%
Cholesterol 209mg 70%
Sodium 1016mg   44%
Total Carbohydrate 19g   7%
Dietary Fiber 0.3g   1%
Total Sugars 11.3g
Protein 53.9g
Vitamin D 0mcg   0%
Calcium 65mg   5%
Iron 3mg   14%
Potassium 911mg   19%

Pork Loin

Cooking Time: 32 Minutes
Yield: 1 Serving
Ingredients
2 cloves of garlic, chopped
½ tablespoon of chopped fresh rosemary
1 tablespoon of olive oil, divided
1 pound of pork loin
Salt, to taste
 Black pepper, to taste
1/8 cup dry white wine
Directions
1. Take a large bowl and add garlic, rosemary and half of olive oil.
2. Insert the tip of the paring knife few times in the top of the pork loin.
3. Fill each opening with herb mixture.
4. Rub it generously so the meat coats well.
5. Now, turn on the sauté mode of the mini instant pot.
6. Add the remaining oil in the instant pot and add pork.
7. Cook the pork until golden brown for about 7 minutes.
8. Now add in the wine.
9. Lock the pot and set the cooking time to 25 minutes at high pressure.
10. Afterward, quick release the steam.
11. Transfer the pork to a cutting board.
12. Let it sit for 5 minutes.
13. Then slice the pork and spoon the juice from the pot on the top.
14. Enjoy with a sprinkle of salt and black pepper.

Nutrition Facts
Servings: 1
Amount per serving
Calories   1257
% Daily Value*
Total Fat 77.4g   99%
Saturated Fat 25.9g 129%
Cholesterol 363mg 121%
Sodium 440mg   19%
Total Carbohydrate 3.9g   1%
Dietary Fiber 0.9g   3%
Total Sugars 0.3g
Protein 124.4g
Vitamin D 0mcg   0%
Calcium 121mg   9%
Iron 5mg   26%
Potassium 1989mg 42%

Mini Pot Roast

Cooking Time: 50 Minutes
Yield: 2 Servings
Ingredients
2 tablespoons of extra-virgin olive oil
1 pound of chuck roast
2 tablespoons butter
1 tablespoon ranch dressing mix, dry
2 tablespoons of dry au jus mix
Black pepper, to taste
Directions
1. Turn on the sauté mode of the mini instant pot and then add oil to it.
2. When the display gives hot, add the roast to the mini instant pot and let it cook for 10 minutes, turn after 5 minutes to cook from both sides.
3. Then turn off the mini instant pot and take out the roast.
4. Now rub the butter, dry au jus and ranch, and dressing mix on the roast.
5. Next, add 1/3 cup of water to the same pot and add the roast to the pot.
6. Then close the lid.
7. Turn on the stew button, and set the timer to 35 minutes.
8. Once the cooking timer beeps, release the steam naturally.
9. Press Cancel and turn off the Instant Pot.
10. Next, open the pot by removing the lid and transfer the meat to an oil greased baking dish.
11. Pour the liquid from the instant pot over the roast.
12. Now broil the meat in the oven at 350 degrees F for 5 minutes.
13. Serve and enjoy.

Nutrition Facts
Servings: 2
Amount per serving
Calories   731
% Daily Value*
Total Fat 44.7g   57%
Saturated Fat 16.2g 81%
Cholesterol 260mg 87%
Sodium 1072mg   47%
Total Carbohydrate 3.9g   1%
Dietary Fiber 0.1g   0%
Total Sugars 0.3g
Protein 75.2g
Vitamin D 8mcg   40%
Calcium 31mg   2%
Iron 9mg   49%
Potassium 660mg   14%

Delicious Pork Recipe

Cooking Time: 50 Minutes
Yield: 1 Serving

Ingredients
4 tablespoons of orange juice
3 tablespoons of lemon juice
2 cloves garlic, minced
Salt, to taste
1 pound grass-fed pork shoulder, cut into 3-inch cubes(boneless)
Fresh cilantro, chopped

Directions
1. Combine the orange juice, lemon juice, salt, garlic and pork inside the pot.
2. Set the timer to 40 minutes and close the lid.
3. After 40 minutes, press the cancel button and allow the steam to release naturally.
4. Preheat the oven broiler.
5. Remove the meat from the pot to the baking sheet.
6. Set the mini instant pot to sauté mode and cook the liquid.
7. Meanwhile, broil the pork meat for 4-5 minutes per side.
8. Once it's crispy take out the pork.
9. Serve it with the drizzle of pot juice.
10. Enjoy.

Nutrition Facts
Servings: 1
Amount per serving
Calories   1114
% Daily Value*
Total Fat 61.7g   79%
Saturated Fat 21.8g 109%
Cholesterol 408mg 136%
Sodium 502mg   22%
Total Carbohydrate 19.7g 7%
Dietary Fiber 1g   3%
Total Sugars 7.5g
Protein 116.3g
Vitamin D 0mcg   0%
Calcium 114mg   9%
Iron 8mg   44%
Potassium 1891mg 40%

Simple Beef Meatballs

Cooking Time: 20-25 Minutes
Yield: 2 Servings

Ingredients
1 pound of lean ground beef
4 tablespoons of   almond flour
2 small eggs
Salt and black pepper, to taste
½ cup tomato sauce
½ cup beef broth

Directions
1. Take a medium bowl and combine almond flour, ground beef, eggs, salt, and pepper.
2. Mix well with hand and make small meatballs.
3. Now pour the broth and tomato sauce into the instant pot.
4. Now add meatball to the pot and stir slightly so that the meatballs coat well.
5. Now close the instant pot and press manual button.
6. Adjust the timer to 20-25 minutes.
7. Once the timer goes off, release the steam naturally.
8. Now spoon out the meatballs and serve with the drizzle of sauce.
9. Serve warm and enjoy.

Nutrition Facts
Servings: 2
Amount per serving
Calories   619
% Daily Value*
Total Fat 27.8g   36%
Saturated Fat 7.3g   37%
Cholesterol 340mg   113%
Sodium 720mg   31%
Total Carbohydrate 8.1g   3%
Dietary Fiber 3.1g   11%
Total Sugars 3.1g
Protein 79.8g
Vitamin D 13mcg   65%
Calcium 33mg   3%
Iron 44mg   245%
Potassium 1218mg 26%

Fresh Onion Beef

Cooking Time: 43 Minutes
Yield: 2 Servings
Ingredients
2 tablespoons of butter
1 sweet onion, thinly sliced
Salt and black pepper, to taste
1 pound of boneless beef tenderloin, cut into small chunks
4 slices of baguette, 1/2 inch thick (from 14-ounce loaf)
½ cup shredded Swiss cheese
1/3 cups water
Directions
1. Turn on the sauté mode of the instant pot and then add butter and onions.
2. Cook the onions for 3 minutes, and then add in the meat.
3. Cook for 7 minutes until golden brown.
4. Now sprinkle salt and pepper.
5. Add in the water and press the cancel button and then set the time to 30 minutes at high pressure by locking the lid of the pot.
6. Once the instant pot timer beeps, turn off the pot and then set it to "keep warm" setting.
7. Meanwhile set the oven to broil and then arrange the baguette slice on a foiled baking sheet.
8. Sprinkle the slices with cheese and then broil for 3 minutes until cheese melts.
9. Take out the baguette slices.
10. Turn off the instant pot and take out the cooked meat.
11. Serve the meat by placing it over the baguette slices. Enjoy.

Nutrition Facts
Servings: 2
Amount per serving
Calories   879
% Daily Value*
Total Fat 41g 53%
Saturated Fat 20.3g 102%
Cholesterol 264mg 88%
Sodium 687mg   30%
Total Carbohydrate 42.8g   16%
Dietary Fiber 2.7g   10%
Total Sugars 4.3g
Protein 81.2g
Vitamin D 20mcg   99%
Calcium 296mg   23%
Iron 7mg   38%
Potassium 997mg   21%

Basic Beef Stew

Cooking Time: 50 Minutes
Yield: 2 Servings

Ingredients
1.5 pounds of stew meat, beef
Salt and black pepper, to taste
1 tablespoon butter
1 tablespoon tomato paste
1/3 cup of carrots
2.5 cups beef flavored broth

Directions
1. Take a large bowl and add the beef to the bowl.
2. Sprinkle salt and pepper on top.
3. Now oil sprays the inner Pot of mini instant pot.
4. Melt butter in the pot by pressing the sauté button.
5. Add the beef to the pot and cook for 5 minutes.
6. Once the meat gets brown, turn off the pot.
7. Next, add the tomato paste and carrots.
8. Pour in the broth and then secure the lid.
9. Select manual to 45 minutes.
10. Once the cooking time completes, release the steam by the natural release method.
11. Serve the stew with boiled rice or your favorite side serving.
12. Enjoy.

Nutrition Facts
Servings: 2
Amount per serving
Calories   938
% Daily Value*
Total Fat 50.4g   65%
Saturated Fat 20.9g 105%
Cholesterol 376mg   125%
Sodium 790mg   34%
Total Carbohydrate 5.8g   2%
Dietary Fiber 0.8g   3%
Total Sugars 3.1g
Protein 108.7g
Vitamin D 4mcg   20%
Calcium 55mg   4%
Iron 13mg   71%
Potassium 1037mg 22%

Pork Shoulders

Cooking Time: 45 Minutes
Yield: 2 Servings

Ingredients
1 tablespoon of butter
1.5 pounds pork shoulder, trimmed and cut in 3 pieces
1 cup chicken broth
1 teaspoon of brown sugar
2 cloves garlic, finely chopped
Salt and black pepper, to taste

Directions
1. Turn on the sauté mode of the instant pot.
2. Melt butter in the pot and then sear the pork meat for 5 minutes from both sides.
3. Press the cancel button.
4. Take a small bowl and then mix broth, brown sugar, garlic, black pepper, and salt.
5. Pour it over the pork.
6. Now secure the lid and then set the pressure valve to the sealing.
7. Now manually cook it on high pressure for 40 minutes.
8. Then select cancel.
9. Release the steam naturally.
10. Open the pot and take out the pork.
11. Shred the meat with the fork and then toss with the liquid from the instant pot.
12. Serve over the bun and enjoy.

Nutrition Facts
Servings: 2
Amount per serving
Calories   1074
% Daily Value*
Total Fat 79.2g   102%
Saturated Fat 30.6g 153%
Cholesterol 321mg   107%
Sodium 655mg   28%
Total Carbohydrate 3g   1%
Dietary Fiber 0.1g   0%
Total Sugars 1.8g
Protein 81.9g
Vitamin D 4mcg   20%
Calcium 95mg   7%
Iron 5mg   27%
Potassium 1239mg 26%

Meat and Potato Gravy

Cooking Time: 50 Minutes
Yield: 2 Servings

Ingredients
2 small onions, chopped
2 tablespoons of vegetable oil
 2 large potatoes, peeled and cubed
1 pound cubed beef tenderloin, cubed
1/3 cup beef broth
Black pepper, to taste
Salt, to taste

Directions
1. Turn on the sauté mode of the instant pot.
2. Add in the oil and sauté the onion for 2 minutes.
3. Then add meat and cook for 7 minutes until brown.
4. Then add potatoes and broth.
5. Next, press the cancel button to stop the sautéing.
6. Now close the lid of the instant Pot and then set the timer to 40 minutes at high.
7. Once cooking timer beeps, release the steam naturally for 10 minutes.
8. Open the mini instant pot and then serve the dish with boiled rice or any of your favorite side serving.
9. Sprinkle salt and pepper for seasoning at the end.

Nutrition Facts
Servings: 2
Amount per serving
Calories   877
% Daily Value*
Total Fat 35g 45%
Saturated Fat 10.7g 54%
Cholesterol 209mg 70%
Sodium 364mg   16%
Total Carbohydrate 64.7g   24%
Dietary Fiber 10.4g 37%
Total Sugars 7.3g
Protein 73.5g
Vitamin D 0mcg   0%
Calcium 87mg   7%
Iron 7mg   37%
Potassium 2449mg 52%

Instant Lamb Roast

Cook Time: 45 Minutes
Yield: 1 Serving

Ingredient
1 pound lamb shoulder
1 tablespoon salad dressing mix
1 tablespoon of ranch dressing mix, dry
½ cup brown gravy mix
1-1/2 cups water

Directions
1. Combine water, gravy mix, ranch mix and dressing mix in a bowl and then rub the lamb shoulder with it.
2. Let it marinate for 20 minutes in the refrigerator.
3. Then dump it into the pot.
4. Close the lid of the pot and then set the timer to 35 minutes.
5. Once the timer beeps, release the steam naturally.
6. Open the pot and take out the meat.
7. Now set the oven to broil and place the meat on the foiled baking sheet.
8. Now cook the meat in the oven and broil it for 5-10 minutes.
9. Serve and enjoy the lamb shoulder by cutting into pieces.
10. Enjoy.

Nutrition Facts
Servings: 1
Amount per serving
Calories   1064
% Daily Value*
Total Fat 39.4g   51%
Saturated Fat 14g   70%
Cholesterol 410mg   137%
Sodium 3101mg   135%
Total Carbohydrate 36.3g   13%
Dietary Fiber 2g   7%
Total Sugars 5.4g
Protein 133.7g
Vitamin D 0mcg   0%
Calcium 172mg   13%
Iron 11mg   64%
Potassium 1648mg 35%

Chapter 8:10 Delicious Soup & Stews Recipes

Classic Pumpkin Soup

Cooking Time: 20 Minutes
Yield: 2Servings
Ingredients
5 cups beef broth
½ pound of pumpkin, peeled, seeds removed
½ pound of chicken
½ cup onion, chopped
Salt and black pepper, to taste
1 cup sour cream
Directions
1. First turn on the sauté mode of the mini instant pot.
2. Grease it with oil spray and then add onions to it
3. Cook for one minute, and then add chicken.
4. Cook until the chicken gets brown.
5. Then add salt, black pepper, and pumpkin.
6. After a few minutes pour in the broth.
7. Turn off the sauté mode, and set the timer to 20 minutes at high.
8. Once done, release the steam naturally.
9. Open the pot and add sour cream.
10. Stir well, then serve hot.
11. Enjoy.

Nutrition Facts
Servings: 2
Amount per serving
Calories   564
% Daily Value*
Total Fat 31.3g   40%
Saturated Fat 17.1g 85%
Cholesterol 138mg 46%
Sodium 2047mg   89%
Total Carbohydrate 19.1g 7%
Dietary Fiber 3.9g   14%
Total Sugars 6.9g
Protein 50.2g
Vitamin D 0mcg   0%
Calcium 208mg   16%
Iron 4mg   22%
Potassium 1170mg 25%

Oats and Tomato Soup

Cooking Time: 8 Minutes
Yield: 2 Servings
Ingredients
6 tomatoes, chopped
1 cup oats
2 tablespoons of olive oil
1 small onion, chopped
5 cups vegetable broth
Salt, to taste
Black pepper, to taste
Directions
1. Turn on the sauté mode of the instant pot and then add oil to the pot.
2. Next, add onions and cook for 2 minutes.
3. Next, add oats and fry for a minute.
4. Then add the tomatoes and mix well.
5. Fry the ingredients for 3 more minutes.
6. Now pour in the broth, salt, and black pepper.
7. Close the lid of the pot and then sets manual to 3 minutes.
8. Next, release steam naturally.
9. Now open the pot and let the soup get cold.
10. Then process the soup in a blender.
11. Now serve the soup hot by reheating it and then serve.
12. Enjoy.

Nutrition Facts
Servings: 2
Amount per serving
Calories   452
% Daily Value*
Total Fat 20.9g   27%
Saturated Fat 3.5g   18%
Cholesterol 0mg   0%
Sodium 2007mg   87%
Total Carbohydrate 47.6g   17%
Dietary Fiber 9.3g   33%
Total Sugars 13.3g
Protein 21.2g
Vitamin D 0mcg   0%
Calcium 91mg   7%
Iron 4mg   23%
Potassium 1590mg   34%

Instant Pot Black Bean Soup

Cook Time: 23 Minutes
Yield: 2 Servings
Ingredients
1 small yellow onion, chopped
2 cloves of garlic
½ cup of black beans
15 ounces of chorizo
6 cups of chicken stock
Directions
1. Grease the instant pot inner pot with oil spray.
2. Chop the onions and garlic.
3. Transfer both ingredients to the instant pot.
4. Turn on the sauté mode of the pot and sauté them with the chorizo.
5. Cook for 3 minutes.
6. Keep stirring so the chorizo would not stick to the bottom of the inner pot.
7. After 3 minutes of cooking, add the rinsed black beans along with the chicken stock.
8. Scrape any stuck on bits of chorizo.
9. Close the lid of your lid, make sure the vent is closed.
10. Press the bean button on the pot and reduce the time to 20 minutes.
11. If the beans are presoaked, then adjust the time to 12 minutes at high pressure.
12. After 20 minutes, release the steam naturally.
13. Serve with favorite side serving and enjoy.

Nutrition Facts
Servings: 2
Amount per serving
Calories   1181
% Daily Value*
Total Fat 83.8g   107%
Saturated Fat 31.2g 156%
Cholesterol 187mg 62%
Sodium 4921mg   214%
Total Carbohydrate 40.7g   15%
Dietary Fiber 8.2g   29%
Total Sugars 4.7g
Protein 64.4g
Vitamin D 0mcg   0%
Calcium 134mg   10%
Iron 6mg   34%
Potassium 1673mg 36%

Potatoes Soup

Cooking Time: 11 Minutes
Yield: 2 Servings
Ingredients
6 ounces bacon, sliced into bite-sized pieces
1/4 medium onion, diced
2 white potatoes, scrubbed and cut into 2-inch pieces
¼ teaspoon salt
¼ teaspoon pepper
5 cups chicken broth
1/4 cup sour cream
Directions
1. Turn on the sauté mode of the instant pot, and when it displays reads "hot "add the bacon pieces and cook for 2 minutes.
2. Press the cancel button and then remove the bacon from the pot.
3. Now drain the fat of bacon from the inner pot and then add onion, potatoes, broth, salt, and pepper.
4. Stir and secure the lid of the pot.
5. Pressure cook for 9 minutes.
6. Once the cooking complete allow the steam to release naturally for 10 minutes.
7. Remove the lid and then add sour cream to the pot.
8. Stir and then serve the soup.
9. Enjoy.

Nutrition Facts
Servings: 2
Amount per serving
Calories   771
% Daily Value*
Total Fat 45.2g   58%
Saturated Fat 16.5g 82%
Cholesterol 106mg 35%
Sodium 4192mg   182%
Total Carbohydrate 39.6g   14%
Dietary Fiber 5.5g   20%
Total Sugars 4.8g
Protein 48.3g
Vitamin D 0mcg   0%
Calcium 90mg   7%
Iron 4mg   21%
Potassium 1928mg 41%

Carrots Soup

Cooking Time: 12 Minutes
Yield: 2 Servings
Ingredients
1 onion, chopped
1 clove of garlic
1 cup carrots cut in cubes
½ cup of coconut milk
4 cups vegetable broth
1 teaspoon salt
½ teaspoon pepper
Directions
1. Grease an instant pot with oil spray.
2. Turn on the sauté mode of the instant pot and cook onion and garlic for 3 minutes.
3. Press the cancel button and then add carrots, milk, and broth.
4. Stir well and secure the lid.
5. Set the timer to 9 minutes at high.
6. Once the cooking time complete, release the steam quickly.
7. Remove the lid.
8. Stir the soup and let it get cold, then blend in a blender for fine consistency.
9. Sprinkle salt and pepper, then serve.
10. Enjoy.
Nutrition Facts
Servings: 2
Amount per serving
Calories   263
% Daily Value*
Total Fat 17.1g   22%
Saturated Fat 13.5g 67%
Cholesterol 0mg   0%
Sodium 2739mg   119%
Total Carbohydrate 16.5g 6%
Dietary Fiber 4g   14%
Total Sugars 8.4g
Protein 12.3g
Vitamin D 0mcg   0%
Calcium 65mg   5%
Iron 2mg   14%
Potassium 840mg   18%

Easy Broccoli Soup

Cooking Time: 8 Minutes
Yield: 2 Servings
Ingredients
2 cups broccoli florets
1 tablespoon of olive oil
Salt, to taste
Black pepper, to taste
2 white onions, chopped
4 cups chicken bone broth with ginger
1 cup heavy cream
Directions
1. Turn on the sauté mode of the instant pot and then add oil when the display reads hot.
2. Add onions and cook for 3 minutes.
3. Then add broccoli florets, broth, salt, and pepper.
4. Cool for one minute and then press cancel.
5. Close the pot and set the timer to 5 minutes at high pressure manually.
6. Afterward, release steam naturally.
7. Open the pot and add heavy cream.
8. Stir to combine well.
9. Serve and enjoy.

Nutrition Facts
Servings: 2
Amount per serving
Calories   822
% Daily Value*
Total Fat 29.6g   38%
Saturated Fat 14.8g 74%
Cholesterol 82mg   27%
Sodium 5175mg   225%
Total Carbohydrate 18g   7%
Dietary Fiber 4.7g   17%
Total Sugars 6.3g
Protein 113g
Vitamin D 31mcg   156%
Calcium 107mg   8%
Iron 1mg   5%
Potassium 494mg   11%

Simple Beef Stew

Cooking Time: 40 Minutes
Yield: 2 Servings

Ingredients

1 pound beef chuck roast, cubed
Black pepper and salt, to taste
1 tablespoon olive oil
1 small onion chopped
1 tablespoon Worcestershire sauce
2 cups of beef broth

Directions

1. Turn on the sauté mode and add oil, then cook onions in it for one minute.
2. Then add meat and cook for 5-8 minutes until brown from all sides.
3. Next, add salt, pepper, Worcestershire sauce and beef broth.
4. Close the lid of the mini Instant Pot.
5. Press the meat/stew button and set the timer for 30 minutes.
6. Cook at high pressure.
7. Once the timer beeps, release the steam naturally.
8. Open the lid and then ladle the stew on to bowl and serve with bread or your favorite side serving.
9. Enjoy.

Nutrition Facts

Servings: 2
Amount per serving
Calories   943
% Daily Value*
Total Fat 71.5g   92%
Saturated Fat 26.5g 133%
Cholesterol 234mg 78%
Sodium 992mg   43%
Total Carbohydrate 5.7g   2%
Dietary Fiber 0.8g   3%
Total Sugars 3.7g
Protein 64.6g
Vitamin D 0mcg   0%
Calcium 47mg   4%
Iron 7mg   42%
Potassium 775mg   16%

Lentil and Vegetable Stew

Cooking Time: 20 Minutes
Yield: 2 Servings

Ingredient

2 tablespoons of vegetable oil
1 cup onion, chopped
1 cup diced tomatoes with liquid
4 zucchinis, chopped
1/3 cup red lentils
Salt and black pepper, to taste
3 cups water

Directions

1. Press the sauté button on the instant pot.
2. Add onions to the pot along with tomatoes and oil.
3. Cook for 5 minutes, and then add the zucchinis and lentils.
4. Pour in the water with seasoning.
5. Press the cancel and then set the timer to 15 minutes at high pressure.
6. Release pressure naturally for 10 minutes.
7. Then serve.

Nutrition Facts

Servings: 2
Amount per serving
Calories   358
% Daily Value*
Total Fat 15.1g   19%
Saturated Fat 2.9g   15%
Cholesterol 0mg   0%
Sodium 215mg   9%
Total Carbohydrate 46.7g   17%
Dietary Fiber 17.6g 63%
Total Sugars 9.9g
Protein 15.6g
Vitamin D 0mcg   0%
Calcium 142mg   11%
Iron 6mg   31%
Potassium 1778mg 38%

Garlicky Chicken Stew

Cooking Time: 37 Minutes
Yield: 2 Servings

Ingredients

1 pound of chicken, cut into pieces
¼ teaspoon sea salt
1 tablespoon of olive oil
10 cloves garlic or more
3 cups chicken stock
8 tablespoons of coconut cream

Directions

1. Turn on the sauté mode of the instant pot and add oil once the display reads hot.
2. Next, add chicken and let it cook for 7 minutes until brown.
3. Then add salt and garlic and cook until aroma comes, now pour in the broth and set timer manually for 25 minutes.
4. Once the timer goes off, allow the steam to release quickly.
5. Now turn again the sauté mode of the instant pot and add coconut cream.
6. Cook for about 5 more minutes.
7. Then serve this thick cream rich stew hot.
8. Enjoy.

Nutrition Facts

Servings: 2
Amount per serving
Calories   577
% Daily Value*
Total Fat 29.1g   37%
Saturated Fat 15.8g 79%
Cholesterol 175mg 58%
Sodium 1534mg   67%
Total Carbohydrate 9.4g   3%
Dietary Fiber 1.6g   6%
Total Sugars 3.2g
Protein 69.1g
Vitamin D 0mcg   0%
Calcium 88mg   7%
Iron 3mg   18%
Potassium 664mg   14%

Root Vegetable Stew

Cooking Time: 30 Minutes
Yield: 2 Servings

Ingredients

2 tablespoons of olive oil
1 pound grass fed Yak, diced
2 parsnips, peeled and chopped
2 yellow onions, chopped
3 cups bone broth
Salt and black pepper, to taste

Directions

1. Heat olive oil in an instant pot by pressing the sauté button.
2. Then add yak and cook it until golden brown.
3. Then add remaining listed ingredients and set the timer to 30 minutes at high.
4. After 30 minutes, release the steam naturally, and then open the pot.
5. Serve the dish warm, enjoy.

Nutrition Facts

Servings: 2
Amount per serving
Calories   1232
% Daily Value*
Total Fat 81.7g   105%
Saturated Fat 28.4g 142%
Cholesterol 265mg 88%
Sodium 5003mg   218%
Total Carbohydrate 76.7g 28%
Dietary Fiber 14.6g 52%
Total Sugars 16.9g
Protein 79.3g
Vitamin D 0mcg   0%
Calcium 274mg   21%
Iron 3mg   17%
Potassium 2105mg 45%

Chapter 9: 10 Flavorful Desserts Recipes

Peanut Butter Fudge

Cooking Time: 1 Minute
Yield: 1 Serving

Ingredients
½ cup chocolate chips
4 ounces cream cheese
1/8 cup stevia
2 tablespoons of peanut butter
¼ teaspoon of vanilla extract

Directions
1. Combine all the ingredients in a mini instant pot and then lock the lid.
2. Set the timer for one minute at high pressure manually.
3. Once the cooking is done, allow it to cool.
4. Stir the mixture by opening the instant pot.
5. Once mixed well allow it to cook for 25 minutes.
6. Serve and enjoy.

Nutrition Facts
Servings: 1
Amount per serving
Calories   1036
% Daily Value*
Total Fat 80.6g   103%
Saturated Fat 45.8g 229%
Cholesterol 144mg 48%
Sodium 549mg   24%
Total Carbohydrate 59.4g 22%
Dietary Fiber 4.8g   17%
Total Sugars 46.6g
Protein 23g
Vitamin D 0mcg   0%
Calcium 251mg   19%
Iron 6mg   35%
Potassium 657mg   14%

Cheesecake Bites

Cooking Time: 15 Minutes
Yield: 1 Serving

Ingredients
8 ounces cream cheese, softened
¼ cup powdered stevia
¼ cup peanut flour
1/8 cup sour cream
1 egg, whisked
½ cup Water

Directions
1. Take a bowl and beat together cream cheese and stevia.
2. Once the smooth paste is formed, fold in the peanut flour and sour cream.
3. Mix well and then add whisked egg.
4. Combine well to form a batter.
5. Now pour this batter into silicon cupcakes.
6. Cove the cupcakes with the foil.
7. Now pour 1/2 cup of water in an instant pot and adjust rack inside the pot.
8. Place the cupcakes on top of the rack.
9. Now adjust the cooking timer to 15 minutes.
10. When the timer beeps, release the steam naturally.
11. Allow the bites to cool completely.
12. Once cool off, serve.

Nutrition Facts
Servings: 1
Amount per serving
Calories   1173
% Daily Value*
Total Fat 102.6g   132%
Saturated Fat 56.8g 284%
Cholesterol 426mg 142%
Sodium 752mg   33%
Total Carbohydrate 26.4g 10%
Dietary Fiber 9.5g   34%
Total Sugars 0.8g
Protein 43.9g
Vitamin D 15mcg   77%
Calcium 320mg   25%
Iron 6mg   36%
Potassium 1186mg 25%

Angel Food Cake

Cooking Time: 40 Minutes
Yield: 1 Serving
Ingredients
½ cup cake flour
Stevia, to taste
Pinch of salt
6 egg whites
½ teaspoon cream of tartar
1 teaspoon Vanilla
Directions
1. Take a small bowl and combine together cake flour, stevia, and salt.
2. Take another bowl and whisk egg whites along with vanilla until foamy.
3. Then add cream of tartar to eggs and mix it well.
4. Beat it with hand beater until foam peaks the top.
5. Now add this mixture to the cake flour mixture.
6. Pour this batter into a small spring form pan. Leave the top space to expand.
7. Now place a steam rack inside a pot and pour a ¾ cup of water.
8. Now place the spring pan on top of the rack and close the lid.
9. Cook for 20 minutes at high pressure. Then manually release the steam.
10. Remove the lid of the pot and then remove the cake with the oven mitts.
11. Now, turn the cake upside down and then place in the spring pan.
12. Now again pour ¾ cup of water to the pot and then adjust the spring pan on top of the rack. Cover and cook about 20 minutes.
13. After the timer beeps, release the steam by using the quick release method.
14. Take out the pan by opening the lid of the pot. Let it get cool down, then serve.

Nutrition Facts
Servings: 1
Amount per serving
Calories   346
% Daily Value*
Total Fat 1g   1%
Saturated Fat 0.1g   1%
Cholesterol 0mg   0%
Sodium 357mg   16%
Total Carbohydrate 50.6g   18%
Dietary Fiber 1.7g   6%
Total Sugars 2.1g
Protein 28.1g
Vitamin D 0mcg   0%
Calcium 24mg   2%
Iron 3mg   18%
Potassium 643mg   14%

Apple Crisps

Cooking Time: 7 Minutes
Yield: 2 Servings

Ingredients
3 medium sized apples, peeled and chopped into chunks
1/4 teaspoon nutmeg
1/4 cup of water
2 tablespoons butter
3/4 cup old-fashioned rolled oats
1/4 cup of flour
Salt, pinch

Directions
1. Dump the apple cubes on the bottom of the instant pot.
2. Now, add nutmeg, and water on top.
3. Take a small bowl and add butter to it.
4. Melt the butter in the microwave for 2 minutes.
5. Then add flour, oat, and salt to the bowl.
6. Drop this mixture on top of the apple inside the pot.
7. Now close the pot and secure the lid.
8. Cook it on high pressure for 7 minutes.
9. Once done, quick release the steam.
10. Serve hot or cold.
11. Enjoy.

Nutrition Facts
Servings: 2
Amount per serving
Calories   335
% Daily Value*
Total Fat 12.8g   16%
Saturated Fat 7.6g   38%
Cholesterol 31mg   10%
Sodium 161mg   7%
Total Carbohydrate 54.8g   20%
Dietary Fiber 9.3g   33%
Total Sugars 25.5g
Protein 3.7g
Vitamin D 8mcg   40%
Calcium 15mg   1%
Iron 18mg   99%
Potassium 368mg   8%

Chocolate Cake

Cooking Time: 6 Minutes
Yield: 1 Serving

Ingredients
1 egg, whisked
2 tablespoons of Olive Oil
4 tablespoons Milk, Raw
4 tablespoons of All Purpose, Unbleached
2 tablespoons of sweetened Cacao Powder
Salt, pinch

Directions
1. Grease the ramekins with oil spray and set aside.
2. Next, pour a cup of water in your instant pot.
3. Adjust the trivet inside the instant pot.
4. Take a bowl and mix all the ingredients in it until finely blended.
5. Pour this prepared mixture into ramekin dishes.
6. Fill just slightly below the top.
7. Place these ramekins inside the Instant Pot on top of the trivet.
8. Now close the lid and set the timer to 6 minutes.
9. Once the timer beeps, release the steam and open the pot.
10. Take out ramekins and let it get cool down.
11. Then serve.

Nutrition Facts
Servings: 1
Amount per serving
Calories   585
% Daily Value*
Total Fat 42g 54%
Saturated Fat 11.2g 56%
Cholesterol 169mg 56%
Sodium 246mg   11%
Total Carbohydrate 55.1g 20%
Dietary Fiber 13.1g 47%
Total Sugars 3.2g
Protein 19.8g
Vitamin D 16mcg   79%
Calcium 142mg   11%
Iron 6mg   35%
Potassium 139mg   3%

Sugar-Free Banana Bread

Cooking Time: 30 Minutes
Yield: 2 Servings

Ingredients

½ cup of butter
2 eggs
3 medium bananas, mashed
1-1/2 cups all-purpose flour
1.5 teaspoons baking soda

Direction

1. Grease a small Bundt pan with oil spray.
2. Now line a parchment paper on the bottom of the Bundt pan.
3. Now pour water about 1/3 cup in the pot and adjust trivet on top.
4. Now combine eggs along with butter and bananas in a bowl and whisk until smooth.
5. Then gently fold in flour and baking soda.
6. Mix to form a batter.
7. Transfer this batter into Bundt pan.
8. Place Bundt pan on top of the trivet.
9. Close the pot and lock the lid.
10. Cook on high for 30 minutes.
11. Once done naturally release the steam.

Nutrition Facts
Servings: 2
Amount per serving
Calories   855
% Daily Value*
Total Fat 51.6g   66%
Saturated Fat 30.8g 154%
Cholesterol 286mg 95%
Sodium 1335mg   58%
Total Carbohydrate 88.5g   32%
Dietary Fiber 6.3g   22%
Total Sugars 22.2g
Protein 14.4g
Vitamin D 47mcg   236%
Calcium 55mg   4%
Iron 4mg   23%
Potassium 773mg   16%

Fruitful Compote

Cooking Time: 6 Minutes
Yield: 1 Serving

Ingredients

1 cup of blueberries
1 teaspoon cinnamon
2 teaspoons of lemon
1 scoop stevia
Salt, pinch
4 tablespoons of water

Directions

1. Combine all the listed ingredients in your mini instant pot.
2. Cook on high pressure for 6 minutes.
3. Once done, release the steam quickly.
4. Open the pot and serve the warm compote.

Nutrition Facts
Servings: 1
Amount per serving
Calories   91
% Daily Value*
Total Fat 0.6g   1%
Saturated Fat 0g   0%
Cholesterol 0mg   0%
Sodium 158mg   7%
Total Carbohydrate 23.7g   9%
Dietary Fiber 5g   18%
Total Sugars 14.7g
Protein 1.3g
Vitamin D 0mcg   0%
Calcium 28mg   2%
Iron 2mg   12%
Potassium 134mg   3%

Orange Bites

Cooking Time: 12 Minutes
Yield: 2 Servings

Ingredients

8 ounces Yellow cake mix
1-2 eggs whisked
1 tablespoon butter
3 ounces cream cheese
2 tablespoons orange zest

Directions

1. Combine cream cheese in a bowl and smooth it out.
2. Next, add orange zest, egg and butter to the mixture and combine well.
3. Now fold in the yellow cake mix.
4. Mix well.
5. Now pour this in an oil greased small cake pan that fits inside the mini instant pot.
6. Now place a rack in an instant pot and pour 1/3 cup of water.
7. Place the cake pan on top of the rack and cover the instant pot.
8. Cover and cook on high for 12 minutes.
9. Once done, quick release the steam and open the pot.
10. Serve and enjoy.

Nutrition Facts
Servings: 2
Amount per serving
Calories   731
% Daily Value*
Total Fat 36.2g   46%
Saturated Fat 15.8g 79%
Cholesterol 157mg 52%
Sodium 947mg   41%
Total Carbohydrate 91.4g   33%
Dietary Fiber 1.9g   7%
Total Sugars 49.5g
Protein 11.5g
Vitamin D 24mcg   122%
Calcium 212mg   16%
Iron 3mg   15%
Potassium 193mg   4%

Simple and Classic Carrot Cake

Cooking Time: 20 Minutes
Yield: 1 Serving
Ingredients
1-1/2 cups plain flour
Pinch of salt
4-6 tablespoons of butter, unsalted   and melted
1 egg, whisked
1 cup almond milk
1 cup carrots, shredded
Directions
1. Adjust the steamer basket inside the top of the instant pot and pour a generous amount of water about a ½ cup.
2. Grease a cake pan with oil spray and set aside.
3. Take a bowl and combine the flour and salt.
4. In a separate bowl, combine butter, whisked eggs, and milk.
5. Pour this mixture into the flour mixture.
6. Fold in shredded carrots.
7. Mix well to form a batter.
8. Pour this batter into a cake pan.
9. Place it on top of the steamer basket.
10. Select the timer to 20 minutes at high pressure.
11. Then, allow the steam to release naturally.
12. Remove the cake from the steamer basket.
13. Let it get cooled down.
14. Serve and enjoy.

Nutrition Facts
Servings: 1
Amount per serving
Calories   1522
% Daily Value*
Total Fat 108.9g   140%
Saturated Fat 81.5g 407%
Cholesterol 286mg 95%
Sodium 658mg   29%
Total Carbohydrate 119.9g 44%
Dietary Fiber 11.4g 41%
Total Sugars 14.1g
Protein 25.3g
Vitamin D 47mcg   236%
Calcium 130mg   10%
Iron 11mg   60%
Potassium 1189mg 25%

Chocolate Fondue with Dipper

Cooking Time: 7 Minutes
Yield: 2-3 Servings

Ingredients

14 ounces of   Dark chocolate
½ cup light cream
2 tablespoons rum
1 cup of whole strawberries

Directions

1. Pour the chocolate and cream in the mini instant pot
2. Close the lid, and set the timer to 7 minutes.
3. Afterward, quick release the steam
4. Transfer the fondue to a bowl and add rum
5. Serve with strawberries
6. Enjoy this simple and sweet treat.

Nutrition Facts
Servings: 3
Amount per serving
Calories   803
% Daily Value*
Total Fat 45.6g   58%
Saturated Fat 31.4g 157%
Cholesterol 53mg   18%
Sodium 112mg   5%
Total Carbohydrate 82.9g   30%
Dietary Fiber 5.5g   20%
Total Sugars 70.5g
Protein 10.9g
Vitamin D 0mcg   0%
Calcium 272mg   21%
Iron 3mg   18%
Potassium 585mg   12%

Chapter 10: 10 Healthy Rice & Beans & Grains Recipes

Cereal Recipe

Cooking Time: 7 Hours
Yield: 1 Serving

Ingredients
1/3 cup steel cut oats
4 tablespoons pearl barley
1/4 cup millet
1 tablespoon of wheat bran
2 cups Water
Salt, pinch
4 tablespoons honey, for serving

Directions
1. Open the mini instant pot and add the first six ingredients to the pot.
2. Now press slow cook and leave the vent open, cook on "more "setting for 7 hours.
3. Once done divide the cereal among serving bowls and top it with the drizzle of honey.

Nutrition Facts
Servings: 1
Amount per serving
Calories   732
% Daily Value*
Total Fat 4.6g   6%
Saturated Fat 0.8g 4%
Cholesterol 0mg   0%
Sodium 181mg   8%
Total Carbohydrate 165.3g 60%
Dietary Fiber 16.5g 59%
Total Sugars 69.7g
Protein 14.9g
Vitamin D 0mcg   0%
Calcium 55mg   4%
Iron 5mg   26%
Potassium 428mg   9%

Tofu Recipe

Cooking Time: 10 Minutes
Yield: 1 Serving

Ingredients
1 onion, chopped
1 tomato, chopped
Salt to taste
Black pepper, to taste
½ cup pasta
1 cup tofu, extra firm
1-2 servings of bouillon paste

Directions
1. Turn on the sauté mode of the instant pot and grease the inner oil with oil spray.
2. Now, add onion to the pot and cook for one minute.
3. Then add tomatoes and let it cook for2 minutes.
4. Then add salt and black pepper.
5. Mix well and add bouillon paste.
6. Add a generous amount of water that covers the ingredients about ½-inch.
7. Now add pasta and tofu.
8. Turn off the sauté mode.
9. Close the pot with lid, and now set the timer to 6 minutes manually.
10. Afterward, release the steam quickly and open the pot.
11. Serve it hot, enjoy.

Nutrition Facts
Servings: 1
Amount per serving
Calories   1343
% Daily Value*
Total Fat 19.6g   25%
Saturated Fat 3.5g 17%
Cholesterol 280mg 93%
Sodium 1393mg   61%
Total Carbohydrate 228.2g 83%
Dietary Fiber 5.4g   19%
Total Sugars 7.8g
Protein 65.8g
Vitamin D 0mcg   0%
Calcium 596mg   46%
Iron 17mg   96%
Potassium 1369mg 29%

Pasta Recipes

Cooking Time: 10 Minutes
Yield: 2 Servings

Ingredients

1 cup pasta, personal choice preferred
1 tablespoon of olive oil
1 onion, diced
2 small tomatoes, chopped
1 teaspoon curry powder
Salt to taste
Black pepper, to taste
1 1/4 cup Water

Directions

1. Turn on the sauté mode of the instant pot and add oil to it once it displays hot.
2. Next, add the onion and sauté for 2 minutes.
3. Now, add tomatoes and fry it until soft.
4. Now, add black pepper and salt along with curry powder.
5. Cook for one minute, and then add pasta along with water.
6. Turn off the sauté mode and then set the timer to 5 minutes at high pressure.
7. Afterward, quick release the steam.
8. Serve hot and enjoy.

Nutrition Facts

Servings: 2
Amount per serving
Calories   1204
% Daily Value*
Total Fat 16.1g   21%
Saturated Fat 2.3g   11%
Cholesterol 280mg   93%
Sodium 188mg   8%
Total Carbohydrate 218.9g 80%
Dietary Fiber 2.3g   8%
Total Sugars 4.7g
Protein 44.9g
Vitamin D 0mcg   0%
Calcium 84mg   6%
Iron 13mg   74%
Potassium 985mg   21%

Cashew Rice

Cooking Time: 15 Minutes
Yield: 2 Servings

Ingredients
2 tablespoons of ghee
1 teaspoon Garam Masala
2 cups rice
2 cups Water
½ onion, sliced
3 tablespoons cashews
Salt to taste
Black pepper, to taste

Directions
1. Turn on the sauté mode of the instant pot and add ghee to it once it displays hot.
2. Next, add the onion and sauté for 2 minutes.
3. Then add Garam Masala, and cook for 1 minute.
4. Now add cashew, salt, and black pepper.
5. Mix gently and then add rice with water.
6. Stir and turn off the sauté mode.
7. Push the rice button and let the instant pot do its work.
8. Next, quick release the steam and then open the pot.
9. Fluff the rice and serve it warm with Greek yogurt as a side serving if liked.

Nutrition Facts
Servings: 2
Amount per serving
Calories   873
% Daily Value*
Total Fat 20g 26%
Saturated Fat 9.4g   47%
Cholesterol 33mg   11%
Sodium 99mg   4%
Total Carbohydrate 154.7g 56%
Dietary Fiber 3.4g   12%
Total Sugars 2g
Protein 15.5g
Vitamin D 0mcg   0%
Calcium 72mg   6%
Iron 9mg   49%
Potassium 329mg   7%

Rice Pudding Recipe

Cooking Time: 12 Minutes
Yield: 1 Serving

Ingredients
½ cup short-grain white rice well rinsed and drained
2.5 cups whole milk
2 tablespoons of sugar
1 pinch salt
1 small egg, beaten, at room temperature
½ ripe mango, peeled and diced

Directions
1. Take an instant pot and combine milk, sugar, rice, and salt.
2. Now secure the lid of the pot.
3. Cook on high for 10 minutes and then release the steam naturally.
4. Temper the egg slowly by adding one cup of hot milky rice to the egg and mixing it gently.
5. Add that egg mixture to the Instant Pot and remember to keep stirring.
6. Now, turn on the sauté mode of the instant pot and cook for 2 minutes.
7. Now take out the pudding and serve it with mango as a topping.

Nutrition Facts
Servings: 1
Amount per serving
Calories   674
% Daily Value*
Total Fat 24.4g   31%
Saturated Fat 12.7g 64%
Cholesterol 199mg 66%
Sodium 453mg   20%
Total Carbohydrate 89.5g 33%
Dietary Fiber 3g   11%
Total Sugars 72.2g
Protein 27.6g
Vitamin D 257mcg   1285%
Calcium 728mg   56%
Iron 6mg   31%
Potassium 1229mg 26%

Hummus

Cooking Time: 35 Minutes
Yield: 1 Serving

Ingredients
½ cup dried chickpeas, rinsed
3 cups Water
4 lemons, juice and zest reserved
1 clove garlic, peeled
2 ounces cooked beets
Salt and black pepper, to taste
½ cup extra-virgin olive oil, or more for serving

Directions
1. Combine chickpeas with water in an instant pot and cook on high for 35 minutes.
2. Once done quick release the steam and open the pot.
3. Rinse the chickpeas under water and let it sit for a few minutes to cool off.
4. Reserve a few tablespoons of liquid from the pot.
5. Next, add lemon zest, pot liquid, Lemon juice, garlic, salt, and pepper to the food processor and blend for a few minutes.
6. Then add cool chickpeas, beets, and process until smooth out.
7. While the blender is running, add half a cup of olive oil and then process until the hummus is smooth.
8. Now spoon out the hummus and drizzle remaining olive oil on top.
9. Enjoy.

Nutrition Facts
Servings: 1
Amount per serving
Calories   1181
% Daily Value*
Total Fat 90.9g   116%
Saturated Fat 12.7g 64%
Cholesterol 0mg   0%
Sodium 94mg   4%
Total Carbohydrate 89g   32%
Dietary Fiber 25.1g 90%
Total Sugars 21g
Protein 23g
Vitamin D 0mcg   0%
Calcium 202mg   16%
Iron 8mg   45%
Potassium 1389mg 30%

Couscous Recipe

Cooking Time: 4 Minutes
Yield: 1 Serving

Ingredients
2 tablespoons olive oil
½ large onion, chopped
1 3/4 cups couscous
1 3/4 cups Water
2 teaspoons salt or to taste
1/2 teaspoon Garam Masala
1 tablespoon lemon juice

Directions
1. Turn on the sauté mode of the instant pot and add olive oil and onions to it.
2. Cook for 2 minutes.
3. Then add water, couscous, Garam Masala, and salt.
4. Stir and cook on high for 2 minutes by sealing the lid of pot tightly.
5. Once the timer beeps, release the steam naturally.
6. Release the steam naturally.
7. Fluff the couscous, and pour in the lemon juice.
8. Serve by mixing well.
9. Enjoy.

Nutrition Facts
Servings: 1
Amount per serving
Calories   1412
% Daily Value*
Total Fat 30.1g   39%
Saturated Fat 4.5g   22%
Cholesterol 0mg   0%
Sodium 4702mg   204%
Total Carbohydrate 241.8g 88%
Dietary Fiber 16.8g   60%
Total Sugars 3.5g
Protein 39.6g
Vitamin D 0mcg   0%
Calcium 106mg   8%
Iron 4mg   20%
Potassium 636mg   14%

Cannellini and Mint Salad

Cooking Time: 10 Minutes
Yield: 1 Serving

Ingredients

½ cup cannellini beans, soaked
2 cups of filtered Water
2 cloves of garlic, smashed
1 hint of vinegar
1 tablespoon of olive oil
Table Salt, to taste
Black Pepper, to taste
¼ cup of mint leaves

Directions

1. Add beans, water, and garlic in instant pot.
2. Close the lid and cook on high pressure for 10 minutes.
3. When the timer beeps, release the steam quickly.
4. Strain the cooked beans well, and then transfer it to the bowl.
5. Add pepper, salt, vinegar, and oil.
6. Mix all the ingredients well, then serve the salad once cool down my add mint leaves.
7. Stir and enjoy.

Nutrition Facts

Servings: 1
Amount per serving
Calories   441
% Daily Value*
Total Fat 15g 19%
Saturated Fat 2.2g 11%
Cholesterol 0mg   0%
Sodium 199mg   9%
Total Carbohydrate 58.2g 21%
Dietary Fiber 24.6g 88%
Total Sugars 2.1g
Protein 22.6g
Vitamin D 0mcg   0%
Calcium 197mg   15%
Iron 10mg   57%
Potassium 1416mg 30%

Carbonara Recipe

Cooking Time: 12 Minutes
Yield: 1 Serving
Ingredients
½ pound of pasta
2 cups of water
2 large eggs
4 ounces bacon pancetta
1 cup Parmesan
Salt, to taste
Black pepper, to taste
Directions
1. Put the pasta into the instant pot along with water and add salt.
2. Close the lid of the pot and set it to 5 minutes manually.
3. Meanwhile, crack the egg in a separate bowl and then add cheese to the bowl along with pepper.
4. Whisk it until it's all mixed well.
5. Cook bacon in a skillet for 4 minutes at medium heat.
6. Once timer of instant pot beeps, release steam naturally.
7. Dump the paste from the instant pot into the skillet.
8. Remove the pan from heat after 2 minutes and add eggs and cheese.
9. Adjust seasoning and stir for 2 minutes.
10. Mix well and serve it.
11. Enjoy.

Nutrition Facts
Servings: 1
Amount per serving
Calories   1504
% Daily Value*
Total Fat 65.2g   84%
Saturated Fat 31.8g 159%
Cholesterol 698mg 233%
Sodium 2528mg   110%
Total Carbohydrate 131g   48%
Dietary Fiber 0g   0%
Total Sugars 0.8g
Protein 104.2g
Vitamin D 35mcg   175%
Calcium 1602mg   123%
Iron 9mg   53%
Potassium 726mg   15%

Instant Pot Vegetable Rice

Cooking Time: 15 Minute
Yield: 2 Servings

Ingredients

2 tablespoons of sesame oil
1 onion
1 cup carrots
1 cup rice, white
¼ cup celery
Salt and black pepper, to taste
2 cups of water

Directions

1. Turn on the sauté mode of the instant pot and add oil along with the onion.
2. Cook for about 2 minutes, and then add the carrots and celery.
3. Cook for 4 minutes and then add water to the pot.
4. Now add rice and put the lid on the instant pot,
5. Set the timer to 15 minutes.
6. Once the timer beeps, open the pot and fluff the rice.
7. Serve hot.

Nutrition Facts
Servings: 2
Amount per serving
Calories   505
% Daily Value*
Total Fat 14.3g   18%
Saturated Fat 2.1g   11%
Cholesterol 0mg   0%
Sodium 62mg   3%
Total Carbohydrate 84.9g   31%
Dietary Fiber 3.9g   14%
Total Sugars 5.3g
Protein 7.8g
Vitamin D 0mcg   0%
Calcium 69mg   5%
Iron 4mg   24%
Potassium 398mg   8%

Chapter 11: 10 Great Appetizers & Snacks Recipes

Little Smokies

Cooking Time: 5 Minute
Yield: 2 Servings

Ingredients
12 ounces Packages Cocktail Sausages
4 ounces Barbecue Sauce
2 tablespoons of Brown Sugar
½ tablespoon of White Vinegar
2 ounces Beer

Directions
1. Open the instant pot and add sausage to it.
2. Then add BBQ sauce, sugar, white vinegar, and beer.
3. Set the pot setting low and pressure cook for 1 minute.
4. Once the timer beeps, natural release the steam for 5 minutes.
5. Then quickly release the steam.
6. Now if the sauce is not thickened enough turn on the sauté mode and re-cook for 4 minutes.
7. Once done serve and enjoy.

Nutrition Facts
Servings: 2
Amount per serving
Calories   1332
% Daily Value*
Total Fat 102.2g   131%
Saturated Fat 42g   210%
Cholesterol 270mg   90%
Sodium 4718mg   205%
Total Carbohydrate 42.4g   15%
Dietary Fiber 0.3g   1%
Total Sugars 29.5g
Protein 60.1g
Vitamin D 0mcg   0%
Calcium 16mg   1%
Iron 7mg   37%
Potassium 140mg   3%

Instant Pot Five Ingredients Salsa

Cooking Time: 25 Minutes
Yield: 2 Servings

Ingredients

2 cups fresh tomatoes
2 green peppers, chopped & diced
4 large yellow onions, chopped & diced
1 cup seeded & chopped jalapeno peppers roasted
1/4 cup vinegar
Salt and black pepper, to taste

Directions

1. Combine all ingredients in the Instant Pot.
2. Cook it on high pressure for 25 minutes.
3. Then use a quick release method.
4. Once done, refrigerate to let it get cold.
5. Then serve.

Nutrition Facts
Servings: 2
Amount per serving
Calories   206
% Daily Value*
Total Fat 1.7g   2%
Saturated Fat 0.2g   1%
Cholesterol 0mg   0%
Sodium 1447mg   63%
Total Carbohydrate 44.9g   16%
Dietary Fiber 12.8g 46%
Total Sugars 22.3g
Protein 6.7g
Vitamin D 0mcg   0%
Calcium 121mg   9%
Iron 3mg   18%
Potassium 1260mg 27%

Bacon Cheeseburger Dip

Cooking Time: 15 Minutes
Yield: 1 Serving

Ingredients

½ pound lean ground beef
4 slices of bacon cut into pieces
5 ounces diced tomatoes
4 ounces cream cheese, cut into cubes
1 cup of tortilla chips
2 tablespoons water

Directions

1. Turn on the sauté mode of instant pot and when it reads hot, add bacon and cook for 2 minutes.
2. Then add the beef by taking out the bacon from the pot.
3. Cook beef for 7 minutes until brown.
4. Now add bacon, water, and cream cheese to the pot.
5. Place lid on top and then turn into sealing.
6. Cook on high pressure for 5 minutes.
7. Release the steam quickly.
8. Stir and then serve with tortilla chips.
9. Enjoy.

Nutrition Facts
Servings: 1
Amount per serving
Calories   1775
% Daily Value*
Total Fat 110.6g   142%
Saturated Fat 43.7g 219%
Cholesterol 411mg   137%
Sodium 2697mg   117%
Total Carbohydrate 79.4g   29%
Dietary Fiber 7.3g   26%
Total Sugars 5g
Protein 115.1g
Vitamin D 0mcg   0%
Calcium 302mg   23%
Iron 48mg   267%
Potassium 2043mg 43%

Jalapeno Hot Popper & Chicken Instant Pot Dip

Cooking Time: 15 Minutes
Yield: 1 Serving

Ingredients

½ pound boneless chicken breast
4 ounces cream cheese
3 ounces cheddar cheese
3/4 cup sour cream
1/4 cup Panko bread crumbs
1/4 cup of water
Salt and black pepper, to taste

Directions

1. Open the pot and add chicken breast, cream cheese, salt, pepper and water in it.
2. Cook for 10 minutes at high pressure.
3. Then release the steam naturally and open the pot.
4. Shred the chicken and then stir in cheddar cheese and sour cream.
5. Now place the mixture into the baking dish and then add Panko bread crumbs on top.
6. Broil for 4 minters in the oven.
7. Then serve and enjoy.

Nutrition Facts
Servings: 1
Amount per serving
Calories   1646
% Daily Value*
Total Fat 122.1g   157%
Saturated Fat 70.3g 352%
Cholesterol 492mg 164%
Sodium 1350mg   59%
Total Carbohydrate 31g   11%
Dietary Fiber 1.3g   4%
Total Sugars 2.6g
Protein 104.4g
Vitamin D 10mcg   51%
Calcium 990mg   76%
Iron 6mg   34%
Potassium 1073mg 23%

Instant Pot Cocktail Weiner

Cooking Time: 2 Minutes
Yield: 1 Serving

Ingredients

4 ounces of cocktail wieners
6 ounces of BBQ sauce
1/3 Cup water
1 tablespoon of Sriracha

Directions

1. Pour the BBQ sauce on the bottom of the pot.
2. Now pour water and then add cocktail wieners and Sriracha sauce.
3. Close the lid.
4. Cook on high pressure for 2 minutes.
5. Now open the pot by releasing the steam by a quick release method.
6. Serve.

Nutrition Facts
Servings: 1
Amount per serving
Calories   746
% Daily Value*
Total Fat 36.5g   47%
Saturated Fat 0g   0%
Cholesterol 68mg   23%
Sodium 4031mg   175%
Total Carbohydrate 88.7g   32%
Dietary Fiber 1.4g   5%
Total Sugars 59.1g
Protein 12g
Vitamin D 0mcg   0%
Calcium 31mg   2%
Iron 1mg   6%
Potassium 355mg   8%

Instant Pot Popcorn

Cooking Time: 4 Minutes
Yield: 1 Serving

Ingredients

1 tablespoon of butter
1-1/2 tablespoon of coconut oil
½ cup of   popcorn kernels

Direction

1. Turn on the sauté mode of the instant pot.
2. Add oil and butter, and allow it to melt.
3. Once it starts to sizzle, add popcorn and stir to coat well.
4. Place the lid of the instant pot on top, so it holds the popcorn instead while popping.
5. Do not lock the lid.
6. When all the popcorn popped.
7. Transfer to serving bowl.
8. Repeat for the next batch.
9. Once all the popcorns are popped, serve.

Nutrition Facts
Servings: 1
Amount per serving
Calories   284
% Daily Value*
Total Fat 27.6g   35%
Saturated Fat 20.1g 100%
Cholesterol 31mg   10%
Sodium 178mg   8%
Total Carbohydrate 9g   3%
Dietary Fiber 1.5g   5%
Total Sugars 0g
Protein 1.1g
Vitamin D 8mcg   40%
Calcium 3mg 0%
Iron 0mg   0%
Potassium 3mg   0%

Easy Bacon Hot Dog Bites

Cooking Time: 8 Minutes
Yield: 1 Serving

Ingredients

200 grams of Hot Dogs
¼ jar of grape jelly
4 tablespoons of cocktail sauce
2 slices of Smoked Bacon

Directions

1. Cut the bacon and hot dogs.
2. Set the hot dogs aside and then turn on the sauté mode.
3. Cook bacon for 3 minutes in the instant pot, and then separates the grease from the pot.
4. Now add hot dog in the pot.
5. Now add jelly and cocktail sauce.
6. Turn off the sauté mode.
7. Now cook it on high pressure for 4 minutes.
8. Then quick release steam.
9. Turn off the pot and transfer it to the serving dish.
10. Enjoy.

Nutrition Facts
Servings: 1
Amount per serving
Calories   935
% Daily Value*
Total Fat 75.5g   97%
Saturated Fat 28.6g 143%
Cholesterol 148mg 49%
Sodium 4039mg   176%
Total Carbohydrate 22.1g   8%
Dietary Fiber 1g   4%
Total Sugars 17.5g
Protein 37.6g
Vitamin D 72mcg   360%
Calcium 33mg   3%
Iron 4mg   24%
Potassium 529mg   11%

Nuts in Instant Pot

Cooking Time: 20 Minutes
Yield: 2 Servings

Ingredients
1 cup pecan halves
4 tablespoons of maple syrup
1/4 Cup water
1/4 tablespoon vanilla extract
1/4 tablespoon cinnamon
1/2 teaspoon nutmeg
1/2 teaspoon salt

Directions
1. Turn on the sauté mode of the instant pot and add pecans, maple syrup, water, vanilla, cinnamon, nutmeg, and salt to it.
2. Sauté the ingredients for a few minutes, once the pecans get tender turn off the sauté mode.
3. Now add water to the pot and select the cooking time to 10 minutes at high pressure
4. Meanwhile, preheat the oven to 350 degrees F.
5. Once the timer beeps, transfer the pecan to the baking sheet.
6. Bake in preheated oven for 3 minutes, then take out and flip to cook from the other side.
7. Now again place it in the oven and cook for the additional 3 minutes.
8. Once done, let it get cool, then serve.

Nutrition Facts
Servings: 2
Amount per serving
Calories   1089
% Daily Value*
Total Fat 100.3g   129%
Saturated Fat 10.2g 51%
Cholesterol 0mg   0%
Sodium 586mg   25%
Total Carbohydrate 48g   17%
Dietary Fiber 15.6g 56%
Total Sugars 29.2g
Protein 15.1g
Vitamin D 0mcg   0%
Calcium 137mg   11%
Iron 4mg   23%
Potassium 670mg   14%

Classic Wings

Cooking Time: 20 Minutes
Yield: 1 Serving

Ingredients

1 pound chicken wings cleaned and halved
¼ cup honey
¼ cup low sodium soy sauce
½ tablespoon vegetable oil
1 clove of garlic, minced

Directions

1. Take a medium bowl, and mix the honey, soy sauce, garlic, and the oil in it.
2. Marinate the chicken in it, for few hours.
3. Now, pour the prepared sauce along with the chicken in the instant pot
4. Cook on high for 20 minutes.
5. Once done, release the steam naturally.
6. Open and serve the chicken.

Nutrition Facts
Servings: 1
Amount per serving
Calories   1671
% Daily Value*
Total Fat 95.1g   122%
Saturated Fat 26.1g 130%
Cholesterol 381mg 127%
Sodium 2501mg   109%
Total Carbohydrate 76.3g 28%
Dietary Fiber 0.7g   3%
Total Sugars 70.7g
Protein 125.6g
Vitamin D 0mcg   0%
Calcium 89mg   7%
Iron 7mg   41%
Potassium 1005mg 21%

Simple Wings

Cooking Time: 25 Minutes
Yield: 1 Serving

Ingredients

1 pound chicken wings
1/3 cup soy sauce
2 tablespoons of honey
¼ teaspoon ground ginger
¼ teaspoon garlic powder
Salt to taste

Directions

1. Combine all the ingredients in an instant pot, and close the lid.
2. Now, set the timer to 15 minutes.
3. Once the timer beeps, quick release steam.
4. Now layer the chicken onto the baking sheet, and bake in oven at 350 degrees F, for 10 minutes.
5. Once the top is browned, serve and enjoy.

Nutrition Facts
Servings: 1
Amount per serving
Calories   1038
% Daily Value*
Total Fat 33.7g   43%
Saturated Fat 9.3g   46%
Cholesterol 404mg   135%
Sodium 5339mg   232%
Total Carbohydrate 41.9g   15%
Dietary Fiber 0.9g   3%
Total Sugars 36.1g
Protein 136.9g
Vitamin D 0mcg   0%
Calcium 88mg   7%
Iron 7mg   41%
Potassium 1322mg 28%

Chapter 12: 10 Graceful Vegan & Vegetarian Recipes

Graceful Vegetarian Recipe

Cooking Time: 12 Minutes
Yield: 2 Servings

Ingredients
1-½ cups vegetable broth
1 cup uncooked white rice, long grain
Salt and black pepper, to taste
2 cups broccoli, florets
1 cup shredded sharp Cheddar cheese ,(vegetarian version)

Directions
1. Grease an instant pot inner pot with oil spray and then add broth, rice, salt, and the paper.
2. Now add in the broccoli and then secure the lid of the instant pot.
3. Set the time manually for 12 minutes on high pressure.
4. Once the timer beeps, quick release the steam.
5. Add in the cheese and stir twice.
6. Serve hot and enjoy.

Nutrition Facts
Servings: 2
Amount per serving
Calories   616
% Daily Value*
Total Fat 20.3g   26%
Saturated Fat 12.3g 61%
Cholesterol 59mg   20%
Sodium 767mg   33%
Total Carbohydrate 81.2g 30%
Dietary Fiber 3.6g   13%
Total Sugars 2.3g
Protein 25.7g
Vitamin D 7mcg   34%
Calcium 481mg   37%
Iron 5mg   29%
Potassium 554mg   12%

Rice & Beans

Cooking Time: 35 Minutes
Yield: 2 Servings

Ingredients

½ cup Red Kidney Beans, dry
1 cup Brown Rice
½ cup Salsa
2 cups Vegetable Broth
½ cups Water
Salt and pepper, to taste
¼ cup of fresh cilantro, chopped

Directions

1. Add dry red beans and rice to the instant pot and then add in the vegetable broth and water.
2. Give it a stir and then add salsa, salt, and pepper.
3. Now close the instant pot and set the timer to 35 minutes on high.
4. Once the cooking is done, release the steam quickly.
5. Garnish with the chopped Cilantro leaves, and serve.

Nutrition Facts
Servings: 2
Amount per serving
Calories   555
% Daily Value*
Total Fat 4.5g   6%
Saturated Fat 1g   5%
Cholesterol 0mg   0%
Sodium 1165mg   51%
Total Carbohydrate 105.6g 38%
Dietary Fiber 11.3g   40%
Total Sugars 3.7g
Protein 23.4g
Vitamin D 0mcg   0%
Calcium 100mg   8%
Iron 6mg   31%
Potassium 1291mg 27%

Zucchini & Tomato

Cooking Time: 10 Minutes
Yield: 1 Serving

Ingredients

1 fresh zucchini, chopped
½ cup fresh cherry tomatoes
1 cup vegetable broth
¼ cup feta cheese, crumbles
Salt and black pepper, to taste
½ tablespoon of garlic powder

Directions

1. Combine all the listed ingredients in the pot and set the timer to 10 minutes at high.
2. Once the timer runs, release the steam naturally.
3. Open the pot and then serve the chunky soup warm.
4. Enjoy.

Nutrition Facts
Servings: 1
Amount per serving
Calories   125
% Daily Value*
Total Fat 3.9g   5%
Saturated Fat 1.6g   8%
Cholesterol 6mg   2%
Sodium 883mg   38%
Total Carbohydrate 14.6g   5%
Dietary Fiber 3.9g   14%
Total Sugars 7.5g
Protein 10.2g
Vitamin D 0mcg   0%
Calcium 89mg   7%
Iron 2mg   9%
Potassium 981mg   21%

Dump Cake

Cooking Time: 25 Minutes
Yield: 2 Servings

Ingredients

1 cup of cake mix
½ can apple pie filling
1 tablespoon butter
1 cup vegan ice cream, personal choice preferred

Directions

1. Melt the butter in a microwave oven and then add to the cake mix.
2. Mix the ingredients well.
3. Let it a bit lumpy.
4. Now pour the pie filling in it and mix well.
5. Now pour 1 cup water in the instant Pot and adjust trivet on top.
6. Place the batter into a heatproof cake pan and adjust on top of the trivet.
7. Set cooking time to 25 minutes.
8. Afterward, release steam naturally.
9. Once done serve it with ice-cream.

Nutrition Facts
Servings: 2
Amount per serving
Calories   635
% Daily Value*
Total Fat 18.7g   24%
Saturated Fat 7.3g   36%
Cholesterol 30mg   10%
Sodium 704mg   31%
Total Carbohydrate 114.5g 42%
Dietary Fiber 2.6g   9%
Total Sugars 74.6g
Protein 5.2g
Vitamin D 4mcg   20%
Calcium 211mg   16%
Iron 2mg   9%
Potassium 236mg   5%

Instant Pot Mushrooms

Cooking Time: 10 Minutes
Yield: 1 serving

Ingredients

4 ounces mushrooms, sliced
½ cup water
1 tablespoon olive oil
2 garlic cloves, minced

Directions

1. Pour water along with mushrooms in an instant pot.
2. Close the lid of the pot and turn the valve to the sealing.
3. Now press the manual button and set the timer to 5 minutes.
4. Once the timer beeps, open the pot by releasing the stem by the quick release method.
5. Drain the mushroom and then return back to the instant pot.
6. Now add olive oil to the pot and mix.
7. Press the sauté function of the pot and let it cook for 3 minutes.
8. Sauté it by string every 30 seconds.
9. Add in the garlic and once the aroma of garlic comes, serve the dish.

Nutrition Facts
Servings: 1
Amount per serving
Calories   153
% Daily Value*
Total Fat 14.4g   18%
Saturated Fat 2g   10%
Cholesterol 0mg   0%
Sodium 11mg   0%
Total Carbohydrate 5.7g   2%
Dietary Fiber 1.3g   5%
Total Sugars 2g
Protein 3.9g
Vitamin D 408mcg   2041%
Calcium 14mg   1%
Iron 3mg   19%
Potassium 386mg   8%

Sweet Potato Curry

Cooking Time: 10 Minutes
Yield: 1 Serving

Ingredients

2 sweet potatoes, peeled and cubed
1 onion, thinly sliced
1 cup of water
1 teaspoon of Curry Powder
2 tablespoons of olive oil
1 tablespoon of brown sugar
Salt and black pepper, to taste

Directions

1. Turn on the sauté mode of the instant pot and then add olive oil to it.
2. Next, add the onion and cook for 2 minutes.
3. Then add curry powder, salt, brown sugar, black pepper, and water.
4. Then add in the sweet potatoes.
5. Close the lid and then cooked for 8 minutes.
6. Once the timer runs off releases the steam naturally and opens the pot.
7. Adjust the salt and then serve.
8. Enjoy.

Nutrition Facts
Servings: 1
Amount per serving
Calories   839
% Daily Value*
Total Fat 27.1g   35%
Saturated Fat 16.2g 81%
Cholesterol 66mg   22%
Sodium 1464mg   64%
Total Carbohydrate 142.9g 52%
Dietary Fiber 16.5g   59%
Total Sugars 18.7g
Protein 12.4g
Vitamin D 0mcg   0%
Calcium 119mg   9%
Iron 4mg   22%
Potassium 2243mg 48%

Cauliflower Recipes

Cooking Time: 10 Minutes
Yield: 1 Serving

Ingredients

1 tablespoon of olive oil
1 small onion, diced
2 teaspoons Garam Masala
1/2 teaspoon salt
Black pepper, to taste
1 cup of tomatoes, chopped
½ small cauliflower head, cut into florets

Directions

1. Turn on the sauté mode of the instant pot and then add olive oil to it.
2. Next, add onions and cook for 2 minutes.
3. Then add Garam Masala along with salt and pepper.
4. Next, add in tomatoes.
5. Cook it for 5 minutes at sauté mode.
6. Next, add the cauliflower florets and pour in ¼ cup of water.
7. Secure the lid of the pot and cook on high for 2 minutes.
8. Next, release the steam naturally.
9. Serve it with hot rice and enjoy.

Nutrition Facts
Servings: 1
Amount per serving
Calories   182
% Daily Value*
Total Fat 14.4g   19%
Saturated Fat 2.1g   10%
Cholesterol 0mg   0%
Sodium 1184mg   51%
Total Carbohydrate 13.9g   5%
Dietary Fiber 3.9g   14%
Total Sugars 7.9g
Protein 2.6g
Vitamin D 0mcg   0%
Calcium 37mg   3%
Iron 1mg   6%
Potassium 550mg   12%

Curried Potato with Carrots

Cooking Time: 7 Minutes
Yield: 1 Serving

Ingredients

1 small onion
2 tomatoes, chopped
1/2 to 1 teaspoon Garam Masala
¾ teaspoon salt
2 medium potatoes, cubed
4 small carrots, peeled and chopped

Directions

1. First, grease an instant pot with an oil spray and sauté the onions in it.
2. Then cook it for 2 minutes.
3. Then add in the tomatoes and let it simmer for 2 minutes.
4. At this stage add salt, Garam Masala, potatoes, and the carrots.
5. Add in 1/3 cup of water and lock the instant pot
6. Secure the lid and pressure cook at high for 3 minutes.
7. Next, release the steam naturally.
8. Serve hot with rice or any other favorite side dish.

Nutrition Facts
Servings: 1
Amount per serving
Calories   448
% Daily Value*
Total Fat 1g   1%
Saturated Fat 0.2g   1%
Cholesterol 0mg   0%
Sodium 1924mg   84%
Total Carbohydrate 102.7g 37%
Dietary Fiber 19.6g 70%
Total Sugars 24.2g
Protein 11.8g
Vitamin D 0mcg   0%
Calcium 146mg   11%
Iron 4mg   21%
Potassium 3059mg 65%

Vegan Mashed Potatoes

Cooking Time: 5 Minutes
Yield: 2 Servings

Ingredients

4 large potatoes, peeled and cubed
2 cloves of garlic
Salt, to taste
Black pepper, to taste
½ cup coconut milk
Pinch of nutmeg
2 cups water

Directions
1. Cube the potatoes and place it in the instant pot along with water and garlic cloves.
2. Cook at high pressure for 5 minutes.
3. Release the pressure after 5 minutes and then transfer the potatoes to a bowl.
4. Drain the liquid and reserve the garlic.
5. Mash the potatoes slightly and let it sit for a few minutes, so the steam escapes.
6. Mash with the reserved garlic.
7. Now add coconut milk and mix in well.
8. Taste and adjust the seasoning by adding salt, nutmeg, and black pepper.
9. Serve and enjoy.

Nutrition Facts
Servings: 2
Amount per serving
Calories   653
% Daily Value*
Total Fat 15.1g   19%
Saturated Fat 12.9g 65%
Cholesterol 0mg   0%
Sodium 138mg   6%
Total Carbohydrate 120.4g 44%
Dietary Fiber 19.1g 68%
Total Sugars 10.6g
Protein 14g
Vitamin D 0mcg   0%
Calcium 89mg   7%
Iron 5mg   27%
Potassium 3177mg 68%

Mini Instant Pot Spanish Brown Rice

Cooking Time: 35 Minutes
Yield: 2 Servings

Ingredients

1 tablespoon of vegetable broth
2 tablespoons of yellow onion
2 cloves of garlic, minced
1-1/4 cup of brown rice, uncooked
5 ounces of canned tomatoes
Salt and black pepper, to taste
1-1/4 cup of water

Directions

1. Grease the instant pot with oil spray.
2. Turn on the sauté mode of the mini instant pot and add garlic, and yellow onion.
3. Sauté for 2 minutes and then add rice along with vegetable broth.
4. Once the aroma comes, add the tomatoes, and season it with the generous amount of salt and black pepper.
5. At this stage, pour the water.
6. Stir all the ingredients well.
7. Now seal the mini instant pot and cook on high pressure for 33 minutes.
8. Once the time of cooking completes, allow the pressure to release naturally.
9. Open the pot and fluff the cooked rice with the fork.
10. Serve onto plates and enjoy.

Nutrition Facts

Servings: 2
Amount per serving
Calories   366
% Daily Value*
Total Fat 2.8g   4%
Saturated Fat 0.5g   3%
Cholesterol 0mg   0%
Sodium 36mg   2%
Total Carbohydrate 77.1g   28%
Dietary Fiber 4.4g   16%
Total Sugars 2.3g
Protein 8.2g
Vitamin D 0mcg   0%

Calcium 50mg   4%
Iron 2mg   11%
Potassium 457mg   10%

Conclusion

Long gone are the days when people have to put effort and spend a lot of time to prepare a meal that they like to enjoy. The mini instant pot is the latest buzzword that is around with its efficient performance.

Unlike the other appliances, the mini instant pot does not strip away the nutrients from food and doesn't take a long period of time to cook a meal. It is a great appliance to cook food in a few minutes without compromising taste and texture. No wonder mini instant pot is here to rule the lives of couples, students, and singles.

For all the busy bees it is a great value for money as it can perform the task of several appliances. You just put the food in the pot and enjoy a hand free cooking. The food that came out tastes great.

Appendix I: Measurement Conversion Table

Measurement	Equivalent
1 Pound(1 lb)	16 Ounces
1 Cup	16 Tablespoons
3/8 Cup	6 Tablespoons
1/3 Cup	5 Tablespoons+1 Tablespoon
¼ Cup	4 Tablespoons
1/8 Cup	2 Tablespoons
1 Tablespoon	2 Teaspoons
½ Cup	8 Tablespoons
2/3 Cup	10 Tablespoons +2 Tablespoons
½ Cup Butter	1 Stick Of Butter

Appendix II: Cooking Timetable of Mini Instant Pot

Items	Cooking Time
Seafood	1-6 Minutes
Rice	15-35 Minutes
Grains	3-30 Minutes
Beans And Lentils	4-20 Minutes
Lamb Meat	15-30 Minutes
Beef Meat	20-35 Minutes
Duck	10-15 Minutes
Vegetables	2-20 Minutes
Fruits	2-6 Minutes
Turkey	7-25 Minutes